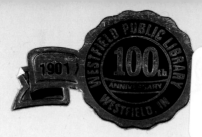

RESTORE
YOURSELF

A Woman's Guide to Reviving Her
Sexual Desire and Passion for Life

RESTORE YOURSELF

A Woman's Guide to Reviving Her
Sexual Desire and Passion for Life

James Simon, M.D.,
and Victoria Houston

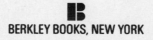
BERKLEY BOOKS, NEW YORK

Every effort has been made to ensure that the information contained in this book is complete and accurate. However, neither the publisher nor the authors is engaged in rendering professional advice or services to the individual reader. The ideas, procedures, or suggestions contained in this book are not intended as a substitute for consulting with your physician. All matters regarding health requires medical supervision. In addition, while the authors have made every attempt to ensure that the information presented is accurate up to the time of publication, medicine is a constantly evolving area of science and ongoing research may lead to changes in some of the concepts presented in this book. Neither the authors nor the publisher shall be liable or responsible for any loss, injury, or damage allegedly arising from any information or suggestion in this book.

A Berkley Book
Published by The Berkley Publishing Group
A division of Penguin Putnam Inc.
375 Hudson Street
New York, New York 10014

PRINTING HISTORY
Berkley trade paperback edition / December 2001

Visit our website at
www.penguinputnam.com

Library of Congress Cataloging-in-Publication Data
Simon, James A.
    Restore yourself : a woman's guide to reviving her sexual desire and passion for life /
James A. Simon and Victoria Houston.
    p.   cm.
    ISBN 0-425-18179-0
    1. Menopause—Hormone therapy.   2. Testosterone—Therapeutic use.   3. Middle aged women—Sexual behavior.   4. Testosterone—Physiological effect.   I. Houston, Victoria, 1945–   II. Title.

RG186 .S6685   2001
618.1'75—dc21
                                                                                2001035407

PRINTED IN THE UNITED STATES OF AMERICA

10   9   8   7   6   5   4   3   2   1

Acknowledgements

A book is never the work of just one or two people. Dr. Simon and I have been blessed with help and inspiration from many directions. First and foremost, we would like to thank the courageous and determined women and men who took the time to share their intimate experiences with us in the spirit of helping others. Without their words, this book would lack authenticity—they give it life.

Among the family and friends whose insights and source recommendations enhanced our work were Debra Simon, Nicole Melcher, Ellen Safire, Carol Davies and Anita Mandl. Professional colleagues without whose help our research and writing might have taken much longer include Carol Mack, M.S.H.S., M.P.H.,

PA-C; Lucy Treen, P.A.; Crystal Claggett, Diana Gould, Mala Prasad and Donna Landis, R.N., C.D.T.; and our transcriber, Sherry Sullivan.

We have been fortunate to have the opportunity to work with Christine Zika, our editor, who enhanced this book with her perceptive editing and excellent suggestions. But we would never have had that opportunity if not for the support of editors Sara Carder and Lisa Considine who guided us along the way. And a warm thank-you to our agent, Martha Millard, who believed in our project from the beginning.

We also gratefully acknowledge the support of Pfizer, Inc.

And, finally, we wish to express our gratitude to Proctor & Gamble and Mary Wulsin for their support of our work with an unrestricted educational grant that made it possible for us to take the time to complete *Restore Yourself*.

Contents

A book about a woman's "male" hormones . . .
Ridiculous! Absurd! Chauvinistic! Well? NOT!

This book is a sincere effort to break new ground and break down old barriers. Its long development (more than six years), illustrates just how hard it can be to gain acceptance for new concepts even when the scientific "facts" have been known for decades.

The book became a reality only because of the persistence of its coauthors and the demographic changes in the world. The idea that a new concept in women's health came about as a result of World War II, and the huge number of postwar "baby boomer" women driving the current economy, seems strangely ironic. But, in fact, that's the way of it. It wasn't until the ranks of menopausal women swelled to more than 20 million, and the potential for commercial success became self-evident, that yet another "hormone book" made it to the shelves. But that's only the tip of the Titanic iceberg and this is NOT just another "hormone book."

As a child of the late sixties, a time I remember most fondly, I recall being struck repeatedly by the similarities rather than by the differences between men and women. One particular experience, which I still recall as if it were yesterday, reminds me of just how similar men and women can be.

It was a beautiful fall day and I was sitting outside the library admiring the fall colors on the surrounding trees when I was drawn to two women walking arm in arm up the path, facing away from me. Both were wearing the standard uniform of the time—tight and tattered bell-bottom blue jeans, custom embroidered. You remember those, don't you?

Each had beautiful reddish-blond wavy hair, about waist length. I recall how stunning their hair was in the sun and even how it matched the leaves still on the trees and those strewn along the ground. I thought to myself how strange it was for these two women to be walking openly, arms linked, on my conservative Midwestern campus. They stopped abruptly when greeted by another acquaintance and much to my amazement, when they turned to face me, one of these "women" had a huge, fluffy, bright red beard, nearly down to *his* belly!

I'll never forget that sight: The young man, ZZ-Topish with his huge red beard, now surprising me with the reality that he was definitely, and I mean *most definitely not a woman*—yet so similar to his companion, a rather attractive woman with equally gorgeous red-blond hair blowing in the fall breeze. How could I have been fooled? Certainly, I know the difference between a man and a woman. Yet from the back, walking arm in arm, I couldn't tell.

This experience has repeated itself numerous times with slight variations. Sometimes it's two women walking together; sometimes it's a man and a woman walking together; and on at least one occasion, it turned out to be two men, even though I thought it was two women. How strange that the visual impression of maleness and femaleness had boiled down to the length of one's hair and the presence or absence of a beard.

Androgyny is a word that means the presence of both gender characteristics. This word epitomizes the importance of this book. My acceptance as a teenager of the commonality rather than the differences between men and women was reemphasized early on in medical school when it became incredibly clear that what I had once thought was a male hormone, testosterone, was in fact also a female hormone.

And what I once thought was a female hormone, estradiol (or a group of female hormones, "the estrogens"), was really also a male hormone. In fact, I was astonished to learn that women make more "male hormone" (testosterone) than "female hormone" (estradiol), and that men make more of both of these during their lives than women! So, which then are "male" hormones and which are "female" hormones?

Another life experience that further convinced me of the importance of both male and female hormones as they relate to an individual's essence occurred during my early professional career when I became Associate Professor of Obstetrics and Gynecology at The Jones Institute of Reproductive Medicine, Medical College of Hampton Roads in Norfolk, Virginia. I had the opportunity to collaborate with a multidisciplinary group of practitioners consisting of gynecologists, urologists, endocrinologists, plastic surgeons, psychiatrists and psychologists.

We were consigned to the Center for Gender Reassignment to work with transsexuals. These were not cross-dressers (transvestites), but rather individuals who firmly believed that they were actually trapped in the body of the opposite sex. Having worked with these individuals over a period of several years, I became convinced that many of them really were men trapped in women's bodies, or women trapped in men's bodies.

Usually, there was no obvious reason for their feelings. It just was the way they were. These were *not* homosexuals. These were individuals who believed heart and soul that they were imprisoned in the body of the opposite gender.

My role in this multidisciplinary group was to provide hormone replacement therapy for these individuals. In other words, I was to give men trapped in women's bodies androgens or testosterone, so that those women's bodies would display the characteristics more commonly attributed to men, with increased muscle mass, lower voices, beards, temporal balding, etc. Conversely, I was to take those women trapped in men's bodies and give them female hormones, estrogens, so that they would look and feel more feminine, with breast development, hip definition, smooth skin, no beards, etc. It was just this experience that convinced me of the extraordinary power of hormones, not only to change the way we look, but also to change the way we feel, and the way we act, and thus further blur what is "male" and "female."

*   *   *

Over the past twenty years I have devoted my career to investigating the similarities, not the differences, between the sexes, as might be determined or predestined by their endogenously produced hormones. Most recently, I have turned the focus of my studies to the investigation of how the absence of one or more of these hormones after menopause may affect a woman's being, and what implications replacement with both estrogens and androgens may have.

Although there have been numerous publications on menopause and hormone replacement therapy, the primary focus of these volumes has been on estrogen replacement therapy, the need for progesterone, and the advisability of utilizing a combination of these. Little has been written about the impact, or in fact, the necessity of androgen replacement therapy in women, as this subject is even more controversial than the issues involved in estrogen or estrogen/progesterone replacement therapies.

I believe that at least one of the reasons for such controversy is our innate ambivalence for, perhaps even fear of, the opposite sex. What man would really want to believe that he makes more "female" hormone than a woman? Or, vice versa, that a woman makes more "male" hormone than "female" hormone? This androgynous fear, akin to homophobia, might be the cause of our reluctance to investigate and prescribe androgens for menopausal women. It is against this background that this book has been written.

My hope is that women will come to know and understand and no longer fear that they, too, have male hormones, and may need to replace them as a result of menopause. Let's even go as far as referring to them all as *human hormones*, without any prejudice or concern about their gender. If our readers can come to recognize and fully accept this intrinsic sameness of all humans, rather than focus so sharply on our differences, then we will have succeeded in our intent.

I would like to dedicate this book to my patients—almost all of whom are women—my mentors, and my daughters. My patients have taught me the importance of being a careful and critical listener. Their stories, many included here (under pseudonyms to protect their identity), are often heart-wrenching. My mentors have taught me that the results of our scientific experiments *never* lie, only that our assumptions and interpretations were wrong. And finally, I would also like to dedicate this book to my three daughters, who will, hopefully, grow and develop in a social climate that celebrates in equal measure the uniqueness of men and women, and the commonality between them.

—James A. Simon, M.D.

Discoveries of fundamental importance may be in store for those who are adventurous enough to leave the safe ground of conventional assumptions and search for newer aspects of reality.
—*Alexis Carrel, 1873–1944*

"Is That All There Is?"
—*song by Peggy Lee*

L ibido. A lovely word. It *rolls* off your tongue: *li-bi-do*. As rhythmic as the act it leads to.

The libido. It arrives without warning, heating our minds and our bodies with desire. It can depart just as suddenly and mysteriously.

My libido vanished in the spring of my 46th year. In turn, I deserted my husband, my lover, the heart of my marriage. I deserted me. Yet I had no idea what was happening, why I was behaving this way.

Even though I was confused, I refused to turn into a dry leaf. It was too soon! I refused to accept reality for one simple reason: I want desire in my life, I want to hold and be held. Luckily, I was not afraid to ask questions. It wasn't easy but I found a way back to the passion that has always been a driving force in my life.

Testosterone. It may sound male—but it is the sweet secret that keeps me feeling like a woman. Here is the story of what I lost and what I discovered. I think this is an important story because it shows that women have a choice. A choice that most of us know little about. A choice that is critical to women today because many of us have men in our lives who—with the advent of drugs like Viagra—have a similar and very potent choice.

My story begins like this: One Sunday morning my husband asked me if I still loved him.

"Don't be silly," I said, busily putting our breakfast dishes in the dishwasher.

"You don't seem very interested in sex," he said. I stopped what I was doing. "You never touch me anymore."

"C'mon," I laughed it off. "I've been really, really busy. You have, too, you know."

"Not that busy," he said as he kissed my cheek lightly and shrugged as if to say he was willing to drop the subject. I made up my mind to stop being so busy. After all, he was nine years younger and the last thing I needed was to feel I was over-the-hill sexually when I most certainly was not. I was busy, busy, busy. And, consequently, very tired at night. I knew that's all it was.

Right? Wrong. But it was going to take me three years to discover what was really happening. Three long years that proved disastrous to what had been a very good marriage.

At the time of this conversation, I was three months away from my regular visit to my ob-gyn. I began to monitor myself and pay serious attention to my own need for physical intimacy. The more aware I became that my husband was right, the more concerned I was—with good reason.

For one thing, I had written a book, *Loving a Younger Man: How Women Are Finding and Enjoying a Better Relationship*, in which I had asserted, based on what I thought was authoritative research, that postmenopausal women rather than feeling less sexy actually feel more sexy because their lower levels of estrogen no longer get in the way of their male hormones like testosterone, which are known to drive our sexual desire. Had I been wrong? The experts wrong? Was I about to prove them wrong?

I went through menopause at the age of 43, which is the norm for women in my family, but early for the general population. Surprising, yes, because you think you have until age 50 or later, but now that the world is finally studying women's health, the medical experts have discovered that many women enter the stages of menopause in their 40s.

That's what happened to me and, on the advice of my female ob-gyn, I immediately started estrogen replacement therapy (HRT) to stave off osteoporosis for which I am at high risk. Could that be the culprit reducing my interest in sex? Or maybe it was just *me*—after all these years of making love, was I bored?

"Sheepish" isn't the word to describe how I felt bringing the subject up with my doctor. "Embarrassed" is more like it. I went over the phrasing of the question for a week before I broached it. Then I rushed my words when I said, "You know, I only ask this because my husband is so much younger but I seem to be less interested in sex these days—is it menopause or the medication?"

My doctor looked at me and gave the question about two seconds of thought.

"It's in your head," she waved her hand dismissively. "You just need to think about it more and use some estrogen cream if you need it. Here, I'll give you a prescription." End of that discussion. I found it curious that she told me the problem was in my head, yet she gave me a prescription for the opposite end.

Okay. I went home and tried to think about "it" more. I pursued all the usual aids. (No, I'm not going to list them—use your imagination.) Result? No major changes in attitude despite the efforts. I could admire my husband's perfect legs one minute and launch a grocery list the next. I began to feel very neuter and not a little depressed by the idea of living the next half of my life feeling unsexy.

Seven months went by. I found myself at lunch with a woman who also has a younger husband and had been a primary source for *Loving a Younger Man*. Diana's husband is fourteen years younger than her and she is in her early 50s. I knew from our interviews that they have always enjoyed a robust sex life. Now she was telling me that she was postmenopausal and had just begun hormone replacement therapy.

Lucky break for me. She is one of the few women I know who is comfortable speaking frankly about her sex life. I asked her the big question: "Have you noticed any change in your interest in sex?"

"I sure did," she announced without hesitation, "and you can be sure that's one thing Hal's not going to put up with. I went right in to my doctor and she prescribed an estrogen combined with testosterone."

"And?"

"Changed my life. No more problems." She smiled happily. "It's a very simple solution."

"What about side effects?" I was skeptical. This must be an outlaw treatment or surely my own female physician would have recommended it.

Diana shook her head and smiled. "I feel great." Two days later she dropped me a note with the correct name of her medication and a copy of a book on estrogen, coauthored by her physician. The book didn't say a great deal about levels of sexual interest but certainly more than I knew about it so far. I was several months away from my annual visit to my doctor. I bided my time, still convinced that Diana's information was questionable and her physician a renegade in the ranks.

Finally it was time for my exam. Midway through, flat on the table in a woman's most vulnerable position, I rushed my words again, saying to my ob-gyn that "I feel fine but I still have this low level of interest in sex and I have a friend who has tried testosterone and . . ."

"Fine. I'll give it to you," said the doctor abruptly. She stood up, whipped off her gloves and started to write on her pad.

"But . . . wait . . . aren't there bad side effects?"

"I don't think so. You'll be fine."

"Well, why didn't you prescribe it before?"

"I make my patients ask twice."

"Why?" I was stunned.

She turned to me with a slight smile. "You never know about the husbands. Many of them are slowing down or they may have problems. Many husbands don't want sex. I don't want to upset the apple cart."

"Oh . . ." I left the office, estrogen/testosterone prescription in hand, mulling over her comment on husbands.

After giving it more thought, my reaction to my doctor's comment escalated to incredulity: *You make a patient wait two years?* You make her conquer the embarrassment of posing the question *twice?* And you never explore with your patient what *her* desired activity level is? Regardless of her husband's situation? What if she's got something going on the side? What if she is widowed or divorced and yearns to have a sexual relationship again? What if she wants to know what *her* options are—not his?

And I had a female doctor. Think how many women have a male ob-gyn and may be too embarrassed to ask—ever!

Later that same week, I had dinner with a woman who is a research ob-gyn affiliated with a large teaching hospital. I'll call her Dr. Number Two. I expected a different answer from Dr. Number Two. She is in her early 30s, and is gay. I expected a stronger advocacy position, I guess.

That is not what I got. First, she interrupted me as I started to describe the loss of my libido.

"Well, of course," she said, "that's perfectly natural. Two years after your last period, you stop producing testosterone—that's why you have no sex drive. Many, many women feel that way." That was a little factoid no one had told me. I hadn't seen that in a book or heard it from my M.D. In fact, that was the very opposite of what I'd been told when researching *Loving a Younger Man*.

I was startled by this news but I also felt better about the problem suddenly. Knowing that I wasn't in a pathetic minority was reassuring. Since then, I've learned that a whopping 70 percent of postmenopausal women may experience a loss of libido.

"Okay—" I told Dr. Number Two the rest of the story and how I was now taking the estrogen/testosterone combination. "Why do you think my doctor didn't tell me this nearly two years ago?" I sputtered.

"We have to be very careful in what we tell our patients," she said after a thoughtful pause. "You see, many women are married to older men and they really don't need to find out what they are missing. If they are happy as they are, why tell them about something that could . . . well, you know."

I was hearing the same thing that the first doctor had told me. I was hearing that the physicians were making judgments affecting a woman's sexuality, her potential for maintaining her normal sex drive, *without informing her of all her options.*

Nor were the physicians taking the time to discuss the options with a couple or learn from them what the two might wish to have happen between them. Instead, the ob-gyns were assuming that most women are with older men (not true, by the way, the U.S. Census showed that 40 percent of women over age 35 are with younger men), that most older men don't want or need to have sex that often and women don't want or need to know that they might have some options, too.

A Woman's Right to Choose

This brings up the old chicken-and-the-egg theory. Which came first? Did she slow down as she hit her 40s and her estrogen/

testosterone levels began to drop? Did he then fall into step with her rather than have family arguments? Would he, could he, perk up if she did? Apparently, if you look at the astonishing sales of Viagra, the drug that helps healthy men overcome impotency, the answer is clear. Yes, men want to have sex. And, yes, they will take a drug that helps them enhance their sexuality.

Other issues can complicate the scene: Is he feeling lower self-esteem because of a career plateau and all the other life changes facing a man in his 40s and 50s? Could that, coupled with his wife's lessening interest in sex, drive him to find appreciation and excitement *outside his marriage*? If his wife can avoid a loss of her libido, perhaps he won't feel that need for sex with another woman.

What if a woman is in a troubled marriage and is planning a divorce? She might like to know that *her loss of libido may not be the result of her relationship with her husband*. What about single women in their 40s and 50s hoping to marry again? Would they opt for an estrogen/testosterone combination that keeps them feeling sexy and exciting?

The essential issues here are the right to information and the right to make our own choices.

Since I began to look deeper into this subject of a woman's libido and how it is affected by an androgen like testosterone in different ways throughout her life, I've learned many surprising things, which we plan to share in the following chapters. My coauthor, Dr. James Simon, is a leader in the medical research being conducted on hormone replacement therapies, including estrogen/testosterone compounds for women.

Of great importance to me—and to you—is that I've learned that the addition of testosterone to my HRT doesn't just enhance my feelings of being a sexually vital woman, but it also has a very positive effect on my heart, my cholesterol levels, my mood and energy levels, my bone density and my cognitive thinking. My entire quality of life as a woman has been markedly improved.

The Testosterone Choice: A New Frontier

So why has so little been said about the specifics of testosterone and the effects it can have on our libido and our lives?

Two reasons. First and most critical, it is a subject most of us are too embarrassed to discuss—among ourselves *and* with our doctors. Those of us, the majority, who see male physicians are in an especially difficult position unless we have that rare doctor who is sensitive to women's self-esteem. Also, a woman may mask her concern over loss of libido by claiming fatigue or depression. Then, rather than respond to a health issue that is a result of hormonal changes, the doctor medicates her for mood swings.

Some women, especially those who live in smaller cities or rural areas, may find the subject socially difficult to bring up with their doctor. One friend of mine put the problem quite succinctly: "My ob-gyn golfs with my father-in-law. Do you think I'm going to ask him why I don't want to have sex?"

The second reason is that the experts are just beginning to more accurately assess the role that androgens, such as testosterone, play in our physical development. The clinical studies under way around the country have only recently reported their test results. They aren't going to have all the answers tomorrow, either. Dr. Simon, whose work continues at the forefront of hormone research, feels the medical community needs at least a decade of research to answer the most important of all the questions.

How This Book Can Help You Choose

That doesn't mean you can't take testosterone if it is a hormone you need and want. It does mean that you need to know the questions the experts are asking. You need to know how testosterone and other androgens are known to work in your body during childhood, adolescence and early adulthood. Then you will better understand what they do as you enter your premenopausal 30s, perimenopausal 40s, during menopause, and when you reach the postmenopausal stage.

In this book we will also discuss the current FDA-approved estrogen/testosterone drugs that are available, as well as those that are in development. You will also be advised on other books and publications about the female body, menopause and estrogen in general, as well as sources for the most current information.

Keep in mind we are all pioneers in this area. Not just the medical scientists making these discoveries, but the women who are finding that we can control our health and our behavior in ways much more beneficial than ever. Our mothers and grandmothers never had access to the medical technology that could delay or defeat osteoporosis and cardiovascular disease the way we do, not to mention adjusting our attitudes and behavior when it comes to sex, a wonderful, enchanting life force we may not want to give up.

In many ways, hormone replacement therapy is at the same stage the science of contraception was twenty years ago. We know some of the benefits, some of the risks. Once you align these benefits and risks against your personal needs, you are in a position to make choices that can improve your life in physically and emotionally satisfying ways. An unexpected side benefit to keep in mind is that because you and your doctor are working with new drugs, you will also find your health being more carefully monitored so you are quite likely to spot unrelated health problems more quickly.

Our physical well-being isn't the only consideration. This book will also help you understand the importance of intimacy in marriage and why that is unlikely to change over time.

Interviews with women who have been taking testosterone for an extended period of time—and a look at an international study of how women feel about the loss of their libido—will explore the emotional issues raised as a woman's level of sexual interest changes. How do husbands feel about this change? How is this likely to affect a marriage or a relationship? Does a woman feel happy or threatened by this change?

How to Use This Book

If the early chapters explain how testosterone is helping women, the latter chapters are designed to help you determine whether or not HRT with testosterone is something you should consider. Chapter Eight features a list of the "most frequently asked questions" that will help you assess your physical symptoms, personal feelings and any emotional issues that may be involved in making this choice.

Not only will this list help you prepare questions that you should ask your doctor before you start estrogen/testosterone hormone therapy, but it will help you decide if the answers are satisfactory or if you should find a better-informed physician.

And for me, personally, what difference has estrogen/testosterone made in my life? Yes, I'm divorced but I have a new and wonderful man in my life. I've recaptured the sweetness and the gentleness that belongs between two people in love. My energy level is high and my health is excellent: I feel terrific. I know this is what is right for me.

I want to help you do what's right for you. I want to give you the confidence to say—the next time *your* doctor or health expert gives you an unsatisfactory answer to a question that has the potential to change your life: "No, that's *not* all there is."

—Victoria Houston

Understanding Testosterone: What It Is, Why We Want It

One

Your First Choice: Listen

Testosterone drives life. This is a fact new to many women. Known as "the male hormone," an androgen, it is too often assumed to exist only in the bodies of men. Not true. As women, we are blessed with "T" from our earliest development in our mothers' wombs. Without testosterone we could not have been conceived; without testosterone, we would never menstruate. Few of us realize that our bodies produce *more* testosterone than estrogen!

"T" is a muted but effective hormone, a ruling force in our own lives, particularly during our teens. Its presence—or lack thereof— can enrich us as we age or leave us feeling barren and bereft. For it is testosterone that incites us to love and romance even as, in later life, it can drive us to push away from the people with whom we once made love. If you are female, you need to know the significance of "T" in your life if only to understand choices open to you today—choices that can change and enrich your life.

Forty-some years ago medical science gave us the Pill, a gift we used to gain control over our lives as women, as mothers, as breadwinners. Now a similar opportunity exists: a chance to restore and maintain the natural balance of our physical chemistry into our middle and later years. This remarkable breakthrough means we have new choices—choices that allow us to restore our love and desire for passion and for life.

A number of women have already begun to make these choices and you will meet them here. Their voices, as well as my voice and the voice of my coauthor, Dr. James A. Simon, are woven throughout this book in order to give you a deeply personal look at how "T" is changing lives.

Starting with me, every woman interviewed for this book has experienced a loss of desire, of libido as well as other symptoms, as a result of a natural or surgical menopause. Several of the women are premenopausal—young women in their thirties—but aware that something was wrong because of their lack of interest in sex. Though other symptoms may have occurred in the lives of each of us, *Restore Yourself* is focused on the loss of libido and other changes affecting our intimate relations with the people we love. It will also examine why each of us feels this is so critical to our lives.

One thing stands out as true of each of the women I've interviewed—we are strong and determined to find our way back to the richness of life as we once knew it. Not one woman in this book found it easy to convince others that something was wrong.

Every one experienced months, often years, of frustration before discovering the benefits of taking testosterone, either alone or with estrogen. These are strong, vibrant, adamant women and we collectively owe them a thank-you—for persevering in their search for physical renewal and for their willingness to share their experiences so everyone who cares will have a choice.

Dr. Simon is a leader in the fields of gynecology, reproductive endocrinology and infertility. He has spent over twenty years in research along the frontier of reproductive endocrinology. In addition to his private practice, he is the president of The Women's Health Research Center; Director of Research for The Osteoporosis Diagnostic and Monitoring Center of Laurel, Maryland; a Clinical Professor of Obstetrics and Gynecology at the George Washington University School of Medicine; and the director of numerous clinical trials of testosterone combinations. Dr. Simon is also a husband, a father to three young women and a careful listener to the women he has treated over the past decade.

While Dr. Simon brings the latest science in women's health to this book, I bring to this book a background of writing on issues affecting women's lives since 1987 and the firsthand experience of being a woman in desperate need of this information. Like many of the women you will hear in these pages, I suffered an immediate postmenopausal lack of libido. Embarrassed and uncertain if it was a physical or emotional issue, I found it very difficult to get good medical advice. Then I had to watch helplessly as the resulting lack of intimacy sabotaged my marriage.

Yet today, eight years after first taking an estrogen-testosterone replacement therapy, I am very happy to report that *I am the woman I was.* I might even be better! I have a rich relationship and a delightful sex life with a wonderful man. Once again I love looking at a guy's legs.

The first of your choices is easy: *listen to us.*

Two

Testosterone: What It Is and How It Works

W hich of the following would you guess to be true of testosterone?

It can A) lift your spirits; B) strengthen your bones; C) reduce
your body fat; D) sharpen your cognitive thinking and improve
your memory; or E) enhance your desire.

If you answered "all of the above"—you are right. Testosterone
is a wonderful hormone, a harbinger of good health physically,
emotionally and intellectually. Much of this information was un-
known a decade ago. Dr. Simon is quick to point out, too, that
even now our scientific understanding of the hormone is still in its
early stages: "For every new answer, we have ten new questions."

Some History on Testosterone

Isolated by a Dutch chemist in 1935, testosterone is closely related to cholesterol in its chemical makeup. It is an androgen, one of the male sex hormones commonly referred to as "steroid hormones." The biologist Adolf Butenandt was the first to successfully isolate testosterone from the testicles of mice. Today it is synthetically manufactured from natural sources—the Chinese cactus, the soybean and the Mexican yam.

Humans produce it naturally—women in their ovaries and adrenal glands, men in their testicles and adrenal glands. The major difference between the sexes is that the average woman will have 40 to 60 nanograms of testosterone in a deciliter of blood plasma, while a man will have 300 to 1000—ten to twenty times more than us girls. It may be known as a "male hormone," but it is crucial to the healthy functioning of the human body *in both sexes.*

Testosterone works in two stages. After conception but before birth, a surge of testosterone is released from the testes of the male fetus to drive the development of a boy child. Meanwhile, the female fetus slumbers on, developing into a girl. The next major surge of testosterone, which occurs in puberty, is systemic—coursing through both the brain and the body—*in both sexes.*

This is news to many women. It is worth taking a detailed look at what occurs during and after puberty because the difference that testosterone makes is delicate and differs with each individual. Understanding the basic chemistry of testosterone will help you understand your body and your self.

*   *   *

Puberty is the dawning of our sexuality, as our sex hormones wake up, pushing our bodies to bloom. Just as boys display body hair, develop upper body strength and experience a rising level of sexual tension, girls are being transformed into women. Exactly how this occurs has only recently been tracked, points out Dr. Simon, noting that it is only within the last few years that medical science has confirmed that a young girl's adrenal glands, not her ovaries, are the first to release her sex hormones.

Released in small doses, these sex hormones charge her brain, becoming evident in early romantic crushes and her first erotic fantasies. This can occur as young as age eight and is followed by activity in the hypothalamus, a neural center in the brain. That action in the brain is believed to trigger—albeit in ways not clearly understood—the ovaries. Now the ovaries take over to become the primary suppliers of the sex hormones.

The body follows the brain: breasts bud, pubic hair becomes evident, fat gathers on the hips, with a growth spurt the pelvis widens and the ovaries prepare to launch the first menstrual flow. And all the while, a young woman is growing more open to erotic thoughts and feelings, fueling her interest and pleasure in things sexual. It is important to emphasize that the sex hormones do not produce behavior. Rather, they heighten her sensitivity to sexual stimulation, enhancing recognition of sexual urges and expressions.

As we move through adolescence and young adulthood, it is the sex hormones that inspire our appreciation of a man's legs, encourage us to cast a meaningful glance, intuitively direct us to stand a little closer and know exactly how to deliver an affectionate touch. And thus—intellectually, emotionally, physically—our libido, the libido of the adult woman, is born.

Orchestrating all this is the hypothalamus, that center at the base of the brain that is now quite receptive to the sex hormones—and quite active in response. And it is this action and reaction that is key to understanding the role of testosterone.

Again, Simon points out, only recently has medical science confirmed that the hypothalamus and the limbic system are the neural centers driving our appetites, whether for food, salt, power or sex. From puberty on, this is the source of our erotic nature. And all because it is receptive to the sex hormones, particularly testosterone. These hormones supply the fuel that makes it operate. Simon believes that if libido starts anywhere, it starts here, and it is greatly affected by our levels of testosterone.

But the science of our libido and our interest in sex is a complicated one, still open to research and questioning. What is known is that testosterone, taken orally, by pellet or skin patch, or injected, does have a direct effect on our libidos. To understand why and how, it is necessary to understand the links between estrogen and testosterone.

Estrogen-Testosterone Links

Estrogen is not a single hormone but a family of hormones, known as the "female hormones." Estrogens are the female equivalent of the male androgens. They are believed to number at least 60 and, like the androgens, exist in both male and female bodies. Women usually have three to ten times more estrogen than men, which is why they claim ownership of this family of hormones. For a wonderful, detailed description of estrogen in all its incarnations, read Natalie Angier's *Woman: An Intimate Geography*.

For our purposes and for ease of understanding the two critical links between testosterone and estrogen, we will discuss estrogen in its primary and best-known form—estradiol.

THE FIRST LINK

The first link between estrogen and testosterone is a simple one: In order to make estrogen, the body needs an enzyme called aromatase. The primary source of postmenopausal estrogens are believed to be testosterone and androstenedione, another androgen that, like testosterone, is generated in the ovaries and adrenals. Aromatase, located in the fat cells, converts these androgens to estrogens. *Thus estrogens begin as androgens.*

How this happens can be best explained with a look at what occurs in early adolescence. As a girl approaches puberty, she and her male counterparts experience a developmental stage called "adrenarche."

Adrenarche is just like it sounds, says Simon. This is the stage in which the adrenal glands are beginning the process of making large amounts of steroid hormones—mostly androgens but these are rapidly converted to both estrogens (including estradiol) and testosterone. Both boys and girls are making bucketloads of both estradiol and testosterone. The only difference is the *ratios* of those steroids.

After adrenarche and a growth spurt, girls go on to begin their

11

menstrual cycles (menarche). And the menstrual cycle is predominantly characterized by fluctuations of estradiol and its sex hormone cousin, progesterone. However, testosterone production in the ovary closely follows estrogen production in the ovary. In fact, it is produced parallel to the estradiol *and in higher amounts*. Except for a few days around ovulation, during most days of a normal menstrual cycle, a woman is making more testosterone than estradiol.

For nearly 70 years, emphasizes Dr. Simon, it has been known that women not only make testosterone, but they make a *lot* of testosterone. In fact, women make more testosterone during a lifetime than they make estradiol.

It is a medical fact that both sexes make both hormones. The differences that distinguish men from women are determined by the ratios of these hormones.

THE SECOND LINK

The second link between testosterone and estrogen is the way they collude to allow estrogen to stimulate our libido.

Most experts in reproductive endocrinology agree that women experience an estrogen "high" at the peak of ovulation and that this is a period of time during which we now know, thanks to numerous studies, that they are more likely to initiate sex.

In her book, *Woman: An Intimate Geography*, Angier cited two studies supporting this. One of lesbian couples, unencumbered with birth control, showed they were 25 percent more likely to initiate sex and had twice as many orgasms during the midpoint of their menstrual cycles than at any other times of the month. In a larger study, 500 women were asked to take their basal temperatures every day for several months. They were to mark down the day of the month when they first noticed an increase in sexual desire. "The pooled results show an extraordinary concordance between the onset of sexual hunger and the time that the basal temperature readings suggest the women were at or nearing ovulation," reported Angier.

Keep in mind, however, Simon cautions, that a woman's androgens, particularly testosterone, spike at this time of the month as well.

So is it the "T" or the "E" working on our libido?

Both and more, says Simon; you can't have one without the other. Here's why: Even as the body produces testosterone and estrogen, it also produces a sex hormone binding globulin that *binds up* some of the estradiol and the testosterone to keep them from reaching the brain. However, these two hormones have opposite effects on this important binding globulin. Testosterone decreases it, allowing more of both testosterone and estrogen to reach the brain; and estradiol increases it, thereby decreasing both estradiol and testosterone's ability to reach the brain and other body tissues. Thus the presence of testosterone makes it possible for some of the estrogens to remain free, reach the brain and stimulate libido. Without the testosterone, the estrogen would be completely bound up and the brain left untouched. No estrogen, no libido.

Concurrent with this, there is some data to suggest that androstenedione (another androgen) is what actually stimulates libido, particularly in teenagers, but also in adults. You'll recall I mentioned earlier that androstenedione is, like testosterone, used by the body's aromatase to produce estrogen. Specifically, testosterone is converted to estradiol, and androstenedione is converted to estradiol's first cousin, estrone. Well, whether it is the testosterone or the androstenedione or their estrogen by-products that have the most direct effect on libido isn't critical to us because we have scientific studies showing that it is the presence of these androgens that *initiate* the effect.

This action becomes clearer when you consider what happens to a woman's body during menopause.

Natural Menopause and Testosterone
(average age 45 to 55)

We now have the research evidence to show that the naturally menopausal woman loses about 90 percent of her estrogen production and about 50 percent of her testosterone production, says Simon. This frustrates other glands, such as the pituitary, that are still attempting to maintain her original menstrual cycle. The result is she has more testosterone relative to estrogen (i.e., estradiol).

So overall the testosterone levels are lower, but the estrogen levels are much lower. A woman's body actually cranks up her testosterone relative to what she had before. Postmenopausal zest—a strong sense of vitality, energy and well-being—may be related to this subtle, relative increase in the level of testosterone.

Meanwhile, the transition from premenopausal hormone production to postmenopausal hormone production in a naturally menopausal woman starts about age 35 and lasts as long as 15 years on average. This long, slow, progressive process is not always completely downhill—it's punctuated by dips and surges. This irregular pattern may even give a woman temporarily *higher* levels of these hormones than she was used to as a much younger woman.

Even though the trend over time is downward, there may be peaks and valleys with peaks higher than those in a normal woman. A perimenopausal woman may experience a period of time when she feels very sexy because she's got tons and tons of estradiol and testosterone on board. Then she may have a menstrual period followed by a cycle during which her body makes very little of either hormone and now she has a dramatic drop in her libido. These wild fluctuations are more the problem in a perimenopausal state than later when the levels are low and absolute.

Even though a woman is losing her testosterone as she reaches menopause, many women who have a natural menopause don't initially have problems with libido unless they're put on hormone replacement therapy. Instead, because of their very low levels of estrogen, they initially have problems with vaginal dryness and pain on intercourse. This leads to a protective mental mechanism. They want to have sex and may even be able to lubricate, but the vaginal tissues may be thinning and easily traumatized. Thus the estrogen deficiency causes a woman to experience pain with intercourse even though she's lubricated. So she gets negative reinforcement for her interest: "I feel sexual but anything I do hurts."

As a result, she may try to overcome this in various ways. She may find herself masturbating away from her partner—this way she doesn't hurt herself—or she and her partner *become sexually distant.* Some couples for whom intercourse is not that important may find satisfaction in mutual masturbation or other sexual activities. That may be fine for some couples but not if their long-term pattern of intimacy has included sexual intercourse. Rather than be frustrated by an increasing lack of closeness in her relationship, she seeks out hormone replacement therapy.

Now an ironic situation develops, says Simon. Before hormone replacement therapy she had more libido, relatively more androgens, relatively more testosterone but not enough estrogen—hence her vaginal dryness. Then her doctor treats her with estrogen—and 90 percent of the time she is treated with an oral estrogen as opposed to a patch. However, one of the consequences of oral estrogen replacement therapy is *it reduces the amount of free testosterone.* (This will be explained in more detail later in this chapter.) Her vagina may be replenished and her lubrication restored but her libido has vanished. Simon points out: She's all dressed up—with no urge to party.

This is exactly what happened to me. I was 43 years old and experiencing vaginal dryness with some pain during intercourse. When I had my hormone levels checked, I learned I was fully menopausal. My ob-gyn recommended hormone replacement therapy—an estrogen/progesterone combination. Just as Simon describes, I was six months into taking the estrogen when I realized my interest in sex was absolutely nonexistent. My body worked fine but my head didn't. As I mentioned in the Introduction, it would be nearly two years before I could convince my doctor to give me an estrogen/testosterone combination that would restore my libido. Meanwhile, my lack of interest in sex had a disastrous effect on my marriage.

Total Testosterone vs. Free Testosterone
and Its Effects

Testosterone and estradiol do not circulate in the blood as free hormones. The overwhelming majority, as much as 99 percent of those two hormones, circulate in the blood bound to a specific protein called sex hormone binding globulin (SHBG) or to albumin. SHBG is a protein made in the liver that binds up the majority of testosterone and estradiol under perimenopausal and postmenopausal conditions. Albumin, a protein present in large amounts in blood, helps in the binding process. That leaves only one percent of the testosterone free to work—to affect libido, for example.

There is one important variation on this theme to keep in mind. When a woman takes oral estrogen replacement therapy, it is delivered via the stomach and the intestines to the liver, stimulating the production of sex hormone binding globulin. In contrast, a nonoral estrogen replacement, such as a patch, goes directly into the blood with less of a direct effect on the liver. This means oral estrogen, which most women take, is likely to result in binding up more of her testosterone, while the patch-type estrogen results in binding up less.

Whichever type of estrogen is being used, the fact is that when a woman has an increase in the sex hormone binding globulin, her free testosterone is decreased. It is further limited because her menopausal ovaries are not able to compensate by producing more either.

The end result is she is now replete with estrogen—hence a

lubricated vagina, a distensible vagina, and less or no pain at intercourse. But now she has little or no libido *because we've bound up most if not all her testosterone*. And there is more happening.

During and after menopause, the pituitary gland tries extra hard to stimulate the ovary, which responds by making some testosterone. In one study Dr. Simon conducted, they learned that when you give estrogen to a postmenopausal woman, whether it's oral or nonoral (also referred to as parenteral), you turn down the pituitary and thereby reduce the drive to the postmenopausal ovary to produce testosterone. A double whammy on testosterone. Not only is more testosterone bound up, but less is produced. Nor is that the end of the story. Simon continues: "For reasons that are unclear, we found that any administration of estrogen, particularly at higher doses, turns off the androgen production from the adrenal glands as well as that from the ovary. So when a woman gets estrogen replacement therapy, at best we turn off her ovaries' production of testosterone. At worst, we turn off her ovaries' production, we bind up what was free, and we turn off her adrenal glands' production. So estrogen therapy can take a woman who felt sexual but had pain with intercourse and make her asexual."

How do we overcome this? A couple of ways. The obvious answer would be to give the woman testosterone—and that does work. But the problem, until very recently, has been that few of the available methods for delivering testosterone to women have been user-friendly. Each has some difficulty involved. Let's look at these.

Options for Increasing Testosterone Levels

The first option is injection. The main advantage to an injection is that the doctor knows when it is given, how much is given, and that it goes directly into the bloodstream. The first difficulty is that the doctor has to do it. The second is that in order to get a relatively stable amount in the blood for a reasonable period of time, such as a month, you have to give too much at the beginning in order to get enough at the end. This carries a risk of side effects, which occur any time that free testosterone levels exceed the normal range. So the primary difficulty with testosterone injections is that you have to "overdose" a woman in order to get enough testosterone to remain in the blood for a reasonable period of time between injections.

A similar option is a subcutaneous testosterone pellet. Same basic difficulties: too much involvement with the doctor as it involves minor office surgery (often not covered by insurance), a period of time where you may overdose, and the necessity to have a compliant patient as regards her estrogen replacement therapy. The latter is important because if she stops taking her estrogen, the relative amount of testosterone will be too high.

Other options include testosterone gels, ointments and sublingual products that can be applied both locally on the genitals and clitoris or can be applied on skin anywhere. The problem with gels, pastes and ointments is that they have a tremendous potential for abuse. It is common for people to believe that if a little is good, a little more is better.

Dr. Simon has witnessed innumerable cases of women who have used these types of testosterone products, increasing their dosage or changing the way they take it, to the point where they have very high levels of testosterone in their blood and significant side effects. Full beards. Balding. Changes in their voice. The loss of subcutaneous fat around the breasts and hips to the point that they look like men. This risk of having superphysiologic levels of testosterone is the drawback to these forms of testosterone.

However, says Simon, there are better alternatives: pills and patches that combine estrogen with a synthetic version of testosterone, known as methyltestosterone. Methyltestosterone is used because it is absorbed better than "plain" testosterone when given orally. Even better than a pill, however, is a new patch (Intrinsa) that delivers testosterone alone or with estradiol, but bypasses the liver. This works better because less testosterone is bound up. The patches are in clinical trials and will be available sometime in the next few years.

Both these options are fundamentally better because the woman can take them without a monthly visit to her physician and the dosages are much lower with a lower risk of side effects. In addition, she now receives the additional benefits of testosterone, which build on the benefits of her estrogen. Studies have shown that adding testosterone promotes bone growth and enhances certain aspects of memory and cognitive functioning, including improved concentration.

Some of testosterone's strongest advocates, including myself, are women who have experienced its absence and its subsequent replacement—and have felt firsthand what a tremendous difference it makes in our everyday, all-around sense of self. We've discovered that a healthy level of testosterone generates a heightened sense of vitality, energy and well-being. Gone are the moodiness, the free-floating anxiety, the unreasonable depression, the insomnia, the fatigue and the lack of focus. Yes, we have our libido back—but our happiness, too.

And these benefits are equally available to the majority of the women who have experienced a surgical menopause as well.

Surgical Menopause and Testosterone
(no average age—can occur in early 20s)

Over 30 million women are surgically menopausal as a result of having their ovaries removed, an oophorectomy. After both ovaries are removed, their testosterone levels will drop by a third or more. The effect of that drop isn't helped by the fact these women tend to be much younger than naturally menopausal women. This makes them more likely to be psychologically unprepared for menopause.

They are tougher to treat because it can be more difficult to separate out the physiologic changes, which include changes in hormone levels, from the psychological changes relating to the surgery or the medical reason for the surgery, said Simon.

And, as he explains, you don't have to have both ovaries removed to experience a surgical menopause. Someone who has just her uterus or just one ovary removed may have similar problems, he said.

Women who have surgical menopause usually are having problems like cancer, abnormal pap smears, fibroids, endometriosis or chronic pelvic pain. When a woman has her uterus removed but not her ovaries, there is the perception that her hormones will be normal after surgery. That may or may not be the case. They need to be tested. Frequently, women who keep their ovaries will find their hormone production is significantly reduced or they may go through menopause as a result of the surgery even if the ovaries were not removed. According to one study, 20 percent of women who have a hysterectomy initially intended to remove only the uterus will still lose function in one of the remaining ovaries or possibly both, as a result of the surgery.

The challenge is that when a woman doesn't have a uterus, she doesn't menstruate so her doctor doesn't know if her hormone levels are normal. "We have to measure them, which isn't easy for several reasons," said Simon. He points out that at the time of their surgery most of these surgically menopausal women are younger and perimenopausal. This makes them moving targets: You measure their hormones one day, their hormones are normal; you measure another day, their hormones are subnormal; you measure a third day, their hormones are supernormal. This is typical of any perimenopausal woman. What do you do? On which set of blood tests do you make your decision?

Then we have more problems. While the actual measuring of the hormones is easy, *interpreting* the results is difficult. First, not all laboratories are capable of measuring estradiol and testosterone accurately in postmenopausal women. In this age of cutting health costs, some laboratories have chosen the "quick and dirty" assays for these hormones. It is important that the physician know how the lab is measuring these levels and that they are accurate.

Second, if the woman really is normal, she's having normal hormonal fluctuations consistent with normal menstrual cycles and normal testosterone production. But if she has a drop in her libido, it isn't necessarily from her hormones. After all, she's had a major medical procedure, a major physical trauma—a hysterectomy.

So not only do you have the effect of general anesthesia and the surgery itself, you have a major psychological effect. She has to accept that this is the end of her fertility, a vital phase of her life. Stress is involved, too. Most women would prefer not to have a hysterectomy or an oophorectomy. She chooses surgery because it's better than dealing with the bleeding or a risky health problem. But given a choice, most women would rather not have the surgery. Her body has forced her to make a decision she really doesn't want.

Simon continues: Now she has lost her reproductive function and our society associates reproductive function with youth—and youth with sexuality. Fair or not, that's the way it is. This makes it hard for a woman who has no uterus to think of herself as youthful and sexy. On top of all that, she wonders if she has a hormonal deficiency. So you can see all the factors at play here.

It can be a very complicated triad between the physical changes that have occurred with the surgery, the hormonal changes that have resulted from the surgery, and the psychological or psycho-social changes that are precipitated.

On the other hand, a surgically menopausal woman is more likely to have a true hormonal deficiency syndrome. Regardless of the exact nature of the surgery, if you measure her hormones and find low levels, it's much easier to convince her that her low libido is a hormonal issue. And once her hormones are replaced, she is very likely to get much better.

Her options are identical to those available to a woman with natural menopause with the exception she may need more hormones, both estrogen and testosterone, because the deficiencies are more pronounced.

Medically Induced Menopause (no average age)

Two categories of medically induced menopause have the same triad of issues as surgical menopause: women who have had pelvic radiation and those who've had chemotherapy.

Radiation is a death knell for the ovaries, explains Simon. They make zero hormone of any kind once they've been irradiated. On occasion the ovaries can be moved out of the way of the radiation with their blood supply (arteries and veins) intact. Then they can be moved back to their proper location once the radiation has been completed. Several experimental procedures have been carried out to have the ovaries "transplanted" to a distant site far away from the radiation beam. These experiments have met with some success. Sometimes, unfortunately, the vagina has also been radiated during treatment. That makes for a more serious problem because even if the hormones are restored, the vagina may not respond to them, instead remaining scarred and nonpliable.

Add to this situation the fact that these brave women have had cancer, a disease that may even be cured but exacts a tremendous emotional toll on the woman and her partner as well. Depression, anxiety and concerns about body image all become important issues, even more so than among women who have lost their uterus or ovaries to benign diseases. Add to that situation a potentially nonusable vagina, despite hormone replacement, and you can see the sexual and relationship problems that may arise.

Simon sees similar problems come up with chemotherapy as women must deal with cancer and issues of death. However, on the plus side, the effects of chemotherapy may not be permanent and its effect on ovarian function may be extremely variable. You can have one 35-year-old woman whose chemotherapy leaves her with no ovarian function at all while another may have totally normal ovarian function even following the same medications. Another will have no ovarian function initially—but that soon changes, and within four to six months ovarian function returns.

The most common cancer and the one presenting the biggest problem relative to hormone replacement is breast cancer. The loss of a breast strikes as devastating a blow to a woman's sense of sexuality as does the loss of her vagina. The breast is incredibly important as a psychological marker of youth and sexuality. The disfigurement that comes from mastectomy and the issue of having a damaged breast, even if it looks normal, is very difficult for many women. Again, this adds a strong psychological overlay to anything biological.

For all these women, the options are dictated by the cancer. For example, women with breast cancer cannot, except under unusual circumstances, use steroid hormones, either estrogens or testosterone. That's loosening up a bit, said Simon, and there are some federally sponsored clinical studies to make sure that our blanket prohibition of estrogen use in breast cancer patients is legitimate. But we don't have an answer yet. We need a good answer to that question because breast cancer is so common.

On the other hand, a woman who has had ovarian cancer, with a few exceptions, is likely to be a good candidate for hormone replacement therapy. Most ovarian cancers are not thought to be hormone dependent, though there are a couple of exceptions. The most obvious is endometrioid carcinoma of the ovaries, but it's rare.

The Perimenopausal Woman and Testosterone
(average age 35 to 50)

Simon is often approached by women frustrated with the wild hormonal fluctuations—and subsequent highs and lows of libido—that occur during the ten to fifteen years prior to menopause. Are these women candidates for estrogen-testosterone hormone replacement therapy?

Sure, he answers, but she is not as quick a study as a woman who is postmenopausal with known low hormone levels. The perimenopausal woman is more difficult to assess because she's a hormonal moving target with hormone levels in constant flux—from high to low to normal. The decision you make on one day is a bad decision for the next day. The goal is to stabilize or minimize these fluctuations. And to do so at the same time you attend to her symptoms. This is not as difficult as it sounds, as you will see in Chapter Three. And a number of pharmaceutical companies are working on medications for the perimenopausal woman with exactly that goal in mind—to stabilize her fluctuations.

Simon continues: Let's look at the problem and how it translates to her libido. The average perimenopausal woman experiencing large fluctuations in her hormones also may have flooding periods, periods with spots and drips only or no periods at all for months at a time. These dramatic fluctuations in bleeding are paralleling dramatic fluctuations in her hormones, both estrogen and testosterone.

You will recall that the hormone levels and the libido cycle together, he points out. So her libido goes up when her testosterone is up; her estrogen is going up when her testosterone is going up. Unfortunately, her bleeding following this cycle goes up when her hormones have been high. So she has high hormone levels, which make her feel sexual. She has sex with her partner and then she has a lot of bleeding. Now she associates the bleeding with having had sex, not with the fact that she's interested—making for negative reinforcement. She decides not to be interested in sex because that's what made her bleed! But the bleeding has nothing whatsoever to do with her sexual activity—it's caused by the increased levels of her hormones. In the end, this interplay takes a toll *on her personal relationship with her partner.*

One simple way to modulate the extremes of her hormones, both highs and lows, is to give her a little bit of estrogen. Or a little bit of estrogen and testosterone. The reason that the latter works is this: Giving her a little bit of estrogen reduces her "thermostat," i.e., her hypothalamus's and pituitary gland's perception that the ovary is not responding. Once the drive to make these excessive levels of hormones is reduced, the ovary follows.

Simon offers an analogy that explains why that happens: If it's wintertime and you've got your thermostat set to 72 degrees, the furnace has to work hard to keep your room at 72. However, if you brought a space heater into the room where the thermostat is and turned it on right underneath the thermostat, the furnace *thinks* that it's warmer than it really is and doesn't work so hard. So if you give a little bit of estrogen to a woman, it turns down her thermostat: It appears that the ovary is making estrogen, but it's not. You're giving a "supplement." Not so much as you get when you take birth control pills, which turns off the whole system. But just enough that the furnace (the ovary) turns on a little less often.

Younger Women and Testosterone (ages 20 and up)

It isn't only women influenced by the symptoms of menopause who experience a loss of libido. Young women taking antidepressants or birth control pills can have this problem.

"I'm often asked if it is possible for women on birth control pills to have decreased libido," says Simon. And the answer is definitely yes—and for the same reasons that women who are given estrogen after menopause may have a decrease in libido.

First, when you give contraceptive hormones to a woman, you turn off her ovaries' production of both estrogen and testosterone. She doesn't ovulate. No eggs. That's the purpose of birth control pills.

Second, birth control pills have a high dose of both estrogen and progesterone or a progesteronelike agent in them. These high levels are required to prevent ovulation. They are all administered orally. Hence, they increase sex hormone binding globulin and bind up the testosterone that's left. So you turn off the source (the ovary), you bind up what's left and you decrease her free testosterone. For some women, this is good. They don't have to worry about pregnancy, their skin is clear and unwanted hair is reduced so they feel more secure and their body image is improved. This is good for sex. Other women, however, experience a decrease in libido in this same setting, despite their improved body image. This is related to the reduction in free testosterone.

In the past 20 years, there has been less and less use of the older androgenic forms of these progesteronelike progestogens in birth control pills—thus fewer side effects. However, in a woman who has a libido problem, the first thing one can do is change to a more androgenic progestogen, which works just like a mild androgen on her sex hormone binding globulin. So a young woman who complains that her libido is low when taking birth control pills may simply need a change in the type of birth control pill she is taking. There may be other causes but this possibility is the first to explore.

This chapter opened with a list of possible answers to the multiple-choice question, "Which of the following would you guess to be true of testosterone?" In addition to answers A through E, one more choice should have been added: "F) It is an option for women of many ages and stages in life."

It is an option, a choice that is changing our lives in deep and satisfying ways. We'll explore just how important this is.

Three

Sweet Libido

T he effect testosterone has on our lives is subtle yet profound. Few of us realize how profound until our testosterone level—*and our libido*—is diminished or has disappeared.

But understanding why our libido is so important to many of us helps us make the choice to increase our testosterone level with a pill, a patch, a pellet or an injection. In this chapter, you will hear the words of other women who are interested in restoring this essential part of our natures.

Their feelings and experiences show that you are not alone in wanting to hold on to this part of yourself. You should not feel embarrassed about it. And you are very likely to gain a new respect for your body and the delicate hormonal chemistry that has driven your life. Once you hear what they have to say, you will understand why the loss of libido was the single most compelling reason that they continued to seek medical help.

How do we know it was low libido that drove them to their doctor's office? Recent medical research shows that when our testosterone levels are low or nonexistent, many of us are likely to experience not only a loss of desire and sexual enjoyment but also depression, anxiety, anger, moodiness, insomnia, fatigue, lack of composure or vitality, memory problems and difficulty concentrating. But in spite of that long list of symptoms, most of the women whose voices grace this book emphasized that the one that pushed them into action was the loss of sexual desire.

Why is this? Why is the loss of libido so important to us that, embarrassed but determined, we seek medical help? And keep seeking it even though the bureaucracy of medical science has not yet recognized female sexual dysfunction—also called FSD—as a health condition that can be officially recognized and pharmaceutically treated? Why do we seek out doctor after doctor, refusing to accept the answer, "It's in your head, nothing you can do about it." Why are we willing to risk hormone replacement therapy when the long-term effects won't be known for years yet?

And if menopause is meant to move us beyond the age of childbearing to a new stage in life, why is maintaining our libido so crucial to us?

One simple reason: sex is not just sex. Sexual intimacy—and the desire that drives that intimacy—is the touchstone of our lives, the bond that connects us to the people we love. From sexual intimacy blooms affection, friendship, understanding, warmth, love and the need to care for one another over the long term. Yes, sex produces babies. But it shapes our natures, too, resonating through the moments and years of our lives, heightening the good days, lighting the dark ones. And it begins deep within us.

"This is who I am at my core," woman after woman said to me as we talked about why they have chosen to take testosterone.

I know exactly what they mean. As someone who lived three years with no libido, refused to take "no" for an answer and opted for testosterone to restore my desire, I know firsthand how testosterone can change your life. When my natural testosterone level dropped it was, at first, the beginning of the end of my marriage. Later, single but with my body and desire restored with an estrogen-testosterone drug, it gave me the option of finding a new partner. Today, I have a wonderful choice to make: I may choose to marry again.

Even if I don't, I am grateful for the gift of my restored libido every morning that I wake and feel the warmth and touch of the man I love. It's an intimacy that reaches far beyond the bedroom— to the kitchen table, to phone calls during the day, to just listening to one another. Not for a moment will I ever take for granted the nuances of our bodies together, the pleasure of wanting and being wanted. I have lived without that and felt empty, dried up, alone. This is how I want to grow old: I love to love and I love to be loved.

But mine is only one voice—here are some others . . .

Celia: The Cost of Intimacy Lost

Blonde, creamy-skinned Celia is soft and lovely at the age of 53. She has a warm smile and a gentle Southern drawl. Like many of us, she didn't recognize the impact that a lack of intimacy could have on her life until she had to live with it.

Five years ago she found herself newly wed to a man incapable of a loving touch, much less sexual passion. The insight did not come overnight but dawned on her over the first year of the marriage, escalating until one day when "I finally realized something was hideously wrong."

A career naturalist and devoted watercolorist, Celia directs the education department for a large zoo in the Midwest. The mother of two adult sons, she left her first marriage in her mid-40s. She sees herself as a woman who has always loved closeness, sex and attention from men, so she was quite surprised when she found herself married to a man who was her opposite. Not only does Celia's story underscore what intimacy *means* to many of us, but it serves as a warning of what can happen when intimacy is *missing*. Her experience mirrors what has been told to me by *men* whose wives are no longer interested in sexual relations.

Celia describes herself as a person who has always had a strong need for intimacy. "It may be my love of nature and the sensuousness of nature that predisposes me to needing intimacy in my life," she says, "but it is important to me to understand things on a very thorough level. And in order to do that, you have to get close. Not just to people but to anything in life. I need intimacy in order to understand and to be happy."

How, then, could she have even been attracted to a man so unlike herself?

Celia reflects on how she made that error. "I've always been a very sexual human being. Sex has been a pleasurable part of my life. I've always had a beautiful body, men have loved my body and I've always felt that any man that I was ever with really got a lot of pleasure from me. Because of that, I have a very healthy sense of myself. And I think I've had healthy sexual relationships with the men with whom I've been intimate. When I met Tom, I made the mistake of assuming that my relationship with him would be as it had always been with a man. When it wasn't, I was surprised. It had a direct effect on my sense of self-esteem, my sense of self."

Still, you ask, how can that happen? Given that they were adults in their 40s who had been previously married, were they not physically intimate before deciding on marriage?

"Our courtship was brief—only six months. Tom had hernia surgery right after I met him, so I just assumed that he didn't want to get involved in anything that might cause discomfort.

"Another thing that should have dawned on me was that there was really no chemistry between us—of a sexual nature. But what was so nice about Tom was that it was so easy to have him in my life. I'd gone back to school for postgrad work. I was completely absorbed, totally focused and loving my classes, the intellectual stimulation. So Tom was great because he was so easy, he made no demands on me. And I thought that was just great . . . at first. It wasn't until later that I realized why he didn't make any demands: He didn't need any kind of intimacy. *He needed nothing from me.*

"But within the first year of our marriage I knew something was dramatically wrong. After I finished my work at the university and had more time for the two of us, I realized how much was missing. So it was near the end of that first year that I realized something was hideously wrong. The second year I tried to figure out what it was and how to fix it . . . but I couldn't fix it.

"I'll give you an idea of what it was like," says Celia. "I could not look into his eyes and have him hold my gaze without his looking away. And I needed to be touched in tender ways once in a while. I needed to be hugged, to be held. But he needed none of those things. For example, he slept in the nude, but if I touched him in bed, he jumped and reacted negatively, not with pleasure. If we were in the kitchen and I hugged him, he would stiffen up and disengage. Usually when you hug somebody, they hug you back so you blend and meld. I never felt that in hugging him. It was always stiff and awkward—he was uncomfortable in an embrace. To me that was weird. I'd never experienced that before. And the last straw was how little we talked.

"So all these little things just added up—the small gestures, the ones that define quality of life and quality of intimacy. I felt deprived of the sensual, simple pleasures of human contact. *The sharing—that's what was missing.*

"I have an analogy that sums it all up," continues Celia. "One thing that attracted me was that I thought we both liked to garden but I have learned there are gardeners and there are gardeners. Tom's gardening style was so different from mine. He wanted all the plants to be separate from each other, where I like plants to blend and mingle and let groundcovers grow and let it be natural. But he wanted everything to be clear-cut and defined and groomed—stand up straight and no dead leaves.

"Even when we were finished working in the garden, he could

never just sit and enjoy it as a pleasure. Instead his mind was always ticking away. 'I've got to transplant that or I've got to prune that.' He was very task oriented, the opposite of a person who could enjoy something just for the pure intrinsic value of being *in it* rather than having to do something *to it*. And that's how he would make love. Mechanically, just like his gardening. It wasn't spontaneous and he didn't seem to enjoy it.

"So now you have two people married to each other who have totally different needs. I could see I would never get what I needed to have. Not because Tom was mean or he didn't care for me. But he did not need, desire or require any kind of real intimacy."

What did she do when she found herself bereft of a closeness she needed so desperately?

"First I thought, 'I do not want to live the rest of my life like this. This is worse than death. I feel like an inanimate object.' Then, of course, I berated myself—why didn't I see this earlier? What was wrong with me? Was I doing something wrong to make him this way? Am I so needy that I need intimacy? That I need to be held? And have it feel good?"

Celia saw a therapist. "She helped me see that the need for intimacy is basic and human. It *is* a natural thing for someone to want. I wasn't at fault—something was indeed wrong. After I told her everything, she said simply, 'I think you know what you need to do.' Her words had a profound effect on me," recalls Celia. "She reaffirmed the importance of my sense of self."

And so the marriage ended. Living without intimacy was a hard, emotionally bruising lesson for Celia. Today she sees genuine intimacy as something that includes sex but also an affectionate touch, a friendly conversation, a meaningful glance. "Intimacy is so important," she says. "I imagine there are people who can have an incredibly sensuous, close relationship without sex, but for me it has been one of the most wonderful pleasures in the world—a vital part of life. *Intimacy is life for me.*"

Celia's story is important for two reasons. First, it shows how her husband's lack of libido—lack of desire for her—resulted in a physical isolation that resonated throughout her entire being. Her loneliness undercut her self-esteem and sense of self.

Second, her feeling that *she was at fault* is one that many men voice whose wives lose interest in sex after menopause. For these men, the loss of physical intimacy reverberates through the marriage and leads to a growing distance between the partners. Unfortunately, most men are reluctant to discuss these issues. Instead, they find themselves in extramarital affairs that restore not only the missing intimacy—but their self-esteem. What is lost is the marriage.

How Women Feel About Menopause and Its Effect on Their Sexuality: "I Don't Want to Lose My Self"

Recently, a major pharmaceutical company working to develop a new testosterone product for women conducted focus groups in the United States and abroad. In one-on-one in-depth interviews with women between the ages of 25 and 60, researchers explored their feelings on menopause and the effect menopause was having on their sexuality. They also explored how the women saw their changing roles as sexual beings and how that, in turn, might affect their lives.

The women were divided into two major sections: naturally postmenopausal and surgically postmenopausal. The latter due to the removal of both ovaries, i.e., "bilaterally oophorectomized."

These two sections were then further divided into three subgroups:

- Women who had "female sexual dysfunction" (FSD) complaints and were not on any type of testosterone therapy or taking any SSRI/antidepressants. They may have been taking estrogen replacement therapy, however;

- Women who had been on testosterone therapy for at least three months;

- Woman who had been taking SSRI/antidepressants.

What they have to say about menopause, loss of libido and the sabotaging of their sexual identity offers more than a window into the heart of a woman—it shows how this core sense of self is vital. Like Celia, these women discover what they are missing when it's gone. Their desperation resonates in the quotes that follow.

ON MENOPAUSE:

"I'm living in someone else's body . . . I'm not a woman anymore . . . I want to go back to the way I was . . . I want to be like I used to be . . . I'm 55—I don't want to feel old . . . I don't feel as connected to my life . . . I'm not as vital . . . I don't have zip . . . I don't have the enthusiasm I used to have . . . I want life to be more fun—more joyous."

ON THE EFFECT OF MENOPAUSE ON THEIR SEXUAL AND
MARITAL RELATIONSHIPS:

"I don't feel as connected—the relationship isn't as vital . . . before we go to sleep there is not the same intimacy as before . . . my husband snuggles but I don't want him near me . . . I've lost my spontaneity . . . life is not as much fun . . ."

ON THE LACK OF ENERGY AND INCREASE IN FATIGUE:

"In the past I was full of power . . . full of energy—now I'm empty and dry . . . in the past I was spontaneous—now it's exhausting to be spontaneous."

ON THEIR TOTAL LACK OF INTEREST IN SEX:

"I have no interest—I wonder if my sex life is finished—will I get it back? . . . I'm not interested in my husband—I have no desire . . . I'm at 'Hi! Don't touch me.' . . . I feel absolutely cold—like a stone . . . on the sexual level, I'm dead—I was not like this before . . ."

ON VAGINAL DRYNESS:

"Sex is painful . . . I experience dryness throughout—my mouth and the sexual parts of my body."

AND ON MEMORY, SLEEP AND CONCENTRATION:

"I used to remember everything—now things just fall out of my head . . . I had a sharp memory—now I write everything down . . . my sleep is very irregular . . . I have a hard time concentrating . . . I am spacey and if I'm pressured, I can't concentrate . . ."

It becomes clear that menopause changes the life of a woman in some pretty incredible ways, ripping apart her sense of self. Those women, many of them younger, who experience menopause as result of a surgical oophorectomy, find the changes especially staggering and are quoted again and again as saying that they "want to restore the desire 'to pounce' . . . to enjoy . . . to desire and relate." Overall, the women reported feeling "betrayed" by their bodies and "desperate."

A summary of comments taken from all the interviews conducted for the study generated this profile of a postmenopausal woman:

- With so few aspects of her "old self" intact, she feels her life is completely out of balance;

- With the disruption of her relationship with her partner and family, she is left with few sources to validate her sense of self-esteem;

- Lacking the energy to go beyond the basic activities and finding herself "shutting down," she no longer feels the freedom to spontaneously enjoy life;

- She experiences so many changes in her body, from mood swings, hot flashes, and energy loss to the loss of sexual desire—that she feels her children, partners and colleagues don't understand her. *She finds her sense of closeness and security threatened in every aspect of her life.*

Some significant differences were noted between the subgroups of women. For example, those who were not on testosterone therapy said they experienced lower levels of energy in general. They also complained that they had lost their desire for sexual contact with their partners, were more easily angered and felt somewhat depressed about their marital relationships. Those who were involved in a sexual relationship with their partner wanted very much to restore their sexual desire and their overall energy level.

Women in the group on estrogen therapy—*but not receiving testosterone*—very explicitly cited their low levels of sexual interest or desire, low levels of sexual arousal and low levels of sexual responsiveness (including orgasm).

In contrast, the women who were surgically menopausal—*and on testosterone therapy*—stated that they perceived themselves to have near-normal sexual interest, sexual arousal and sexual satisfaction.

A major theme through all the interviews was the desire to regain the spontaneity the women had previously felt in their sexual relationships with their partners. Also, one overall opinion was agreed upon by all: the women felt that a more normal sexual relationship with desire, arousal, responsiveness and satisfaction would not only contribute significantly to the quality of their marital relationships, *but it would enhance their general sense of well-being, security and self-esteem.*

The Reality of Testosterone: Sheila and Lauren

To further explore this need for intimacy and how our sexual lives are affected and enhanced when we can enjoy making love, let's look at the experiences of two women, eleven years apart in age, both in long-term marriages and both taking testosterone. Sheila, age 58, has experienced both a natural and a surgical menopause, while Lauren, age 47, has not yet entered menopause. Their individual stories of the loss and restoration of physical intimacy illuminate the value of intimacy in our day-to-day lives.

Petite, lush, silver-blonde Sheila is gifted with an exuberant personality. Her willingness to discuss her sex life saved mine as it was Sheila who introduced me to testosterone. About eight years before she entered menopause, I had interviewed her for another book I was working on. I knew from our earlier interviews and resulting friendship that her marriage of 22 years was thriving, not the least because she and her husband shared a robust sex life. Well-read and health-conscious, she was prepared for menopause and alert to early signs. During a friendly visit, we discussed our mutual experiences with menopause and I asked if she had noted any loss of libido.

"Yes," she answered, adding with a laugh, "and I couldn't let that happen, could I?"

"What did you do?" I asked.

And that was the first I learned of testosterone. Days later, my doctor grudgingly prescribed for me the estrogen/testosterone drug Estratest, which Sheila had recommended, and my life was changed.

A few years after that conversation, Sheila learned she needed a complete hysterectomy as well as the removal of both ovaries, speeding up what had been a natural transition over time to one that was complete overnight. And just as she was coming to terms with all the changes in her own body, her husband faced an unexpected health crisis. Suddenly, two people who had always shared a healthy sex life found themselves separated by health issues that made having sex difficult. These experiences brought into sharp focus the role that desire and sexual intimacy played in their relationship.

"We've always been very physical," said Sheila, "for example, Ben doesn't ask about my day. What he will do is come up behind me and hold me and feel my body. He's much more tactile in that way. And he'll say, 'What's bothering you?' He can tell by feeling."

It was Ben who noticed Sheila's drop in libido shortly after she entered menopause. "This was eight years ago, long before my surgery," said Sheila. "What happened was that all of a sudden I was responding but I wasn't initiating. This was different for me. Through all the earlier years of our marriage, I would often initiate sex—maybe 30–40 percent of the time. And that was completely gone. Ben noticed and he mentioned it to me.

"I realized after he said something that he was right. I felt like I was dwindling away. It wasn't just that I was no longer initiating stuff, but I'd no longer daydream even. It used to be that I'd be walking down the street and think about how I'd like to make love . . . you know, I'd see somebody with a great pair of jeans on and think, 'I'd really like to get some.' That was me. I call it daydreaming, fantasizing, whatever you want to call it.

"Right away I thought it was hormonal and that I would see my doctor about it."

Sheila was fortunate. Her ob-gyn was involved in research on estrogen and testosterone and was already a strong believer in prescribing both. After blood tests to determine Sheila's hormone levels, she prescribed Estratest. Later, after her hysterectomy and the removal of her ovaries, Sheila's prescription was changed to an estrogen patch with a testosterone compound, which she takes sublingually.

"My doctor felt the patch was better because it bypassed the liver and would be safer in the long run. And because of my hysterectomy, I no longer need to take progesterone. Also, it was easy, just once a week. I'm guessing I've been using it three or four years now. It doesn't come off. You pull off a swimsuit and it stays. I wear it on my buttocks, which I prefer to putting it on my abdomen."

After Sheila's surgery, her recovery was complicated and the sheer physical discomfort that resulted made it difficult to resume having sex with her husband. "We had a hard time," she recalls. "We lost a lot of intimacy because Ben literally had to sleep in another room. That's how I realized that for me—and for Ben—

the relationship between intimacy and sex is a very necessary and deep component of our marriage. When Ben could finally share a bed with me and we started to resume intimacy, I found my reaction interesting. When he first moved back into my bedroom, I didn't want him there. I had gotten very used to being on my own and too territorial. Like I wanted the window open, he wanted it closed; I wanted the lights off when I was watching certain shows on TV—I had to hold my tongue a number of times. So that was a problem and it took a couple weeks for me to get beyond that."

Sheila's response to Ben is typical of women with postmenopausal, low testosterone levels. Many women who were previously demonstrative and physically affectionate in sexual and nonsexual ways change as their hormone levels drop; they develop an aversion to their partner's closeness or touch. "It's almost primal," said one woman. "I didn't want him near me." Sheila knew better than to let those feelings continue. Even though her immediate response to Ben's presence in her bed was "territorial," she knew that wasn't what either of them wanted from their marriage.

"To get through that stage, we started what I call 'scx play' as opposed to 'sexual intercourse' and that to me is what the intimacy is all about. We try to do this every day—touch each other in a sensual, sexual way even if we don't have intercourse—in order to have intimacy. During my recovery, I realized I didn't want to lose that. I might have had no sex drive, but I had a tremendous need for intimacy. During that time, of course, I was not taking testosterone. It took us a couple of weeks to get to the point where I felt comfortable having intercourse, which we did. After that, things worked out pretty well. When I was comfortable being intimate and could see myself having sex regularly, I started back taking testosterone.

"Today I take it sublingually," she says. "It's a little chew that comes in different flavors and I get cherry. I think it's cute—like cherry and sex is like a cute little thing to do. There's no brand name. It's just called 'testosterone sublingual zero point one.' My doctor phones it in to a special pharmacy. But it is a controlled substance, which means I have to call my doctor every month."

Sheila's sublingual testosterone enters her system right away. She likes that because "You don't have to take it every day. If you're going away for a weekend and you want to take it, fine; but if you're on your own and not interested in having a sex drive, don't take it." She has had no side effects with the exception of a random coarse hair or two that she plucks immediately. One positive side effect has been an enhanced sense of well-being or, as she says, "I find myself feeling so good when I take testosterone."

But just as they resumed their sex life, Ben got news that he would have to take chemotherapy for a year. Suddenly they could not and would not be having sex. Sheila put away the testosterone.

Again the lack of sexual intimacy challenged their relationship. "Part of my discussion with Ben was I don't want this to become a way of life. I'm not willing to have a celibate marriage; he isn't either. Intimacy does an awful lot to make up for the lack of sex. Believe me, if Ben were having sex elsewhere I'd have a different issue with it.

"But what we have realized is that for us our sexuality and our intimacy is intertwined. So when we don't have sex that whole balance goes out of whack. That's why we've focused on the sex play. It helps us to stay there, to stay connected," said Sheila.

Ben has since recovered and sexual intercourse is once again a part of their lives. Now, however, Sheila recognizes how central it is to their mutual happiness. "What has become very real to me after 22 years is that I took the structure that supported our intimacy for granted. Now I see the threat that a lack of sexual relations can be to our relationship. I'm acutely aware of it. With my health back, I'm very threatened by not having sex. And I've said this to Ben: 'I want you to want me. I don't necessarily want to make love to you. But I want you to want to make love to me. *I want to feel desired.*'

"What I know today is that I need very much to feel like I'm a sexual being who is desired and wanted even if we're not going to be having sexual intercourse. He does, too. He needs the very same thing."

Sheila is 58 years old with 22 years of marriage behind her. She has had wonderful times and years to learn the value of intimacy in her life. Does the same hold true for a much younger woman? For a younger marriage? Is it possible for a woman who has not entered menopause to experience low libido?

Lauren is 47 years old. A slender wisp of a woman whose wide-set luminous eyes, porcelain skin and long, straight blonde hair make her more resemble Alice in Wonderland than a tough-minded tax attorney. Married 16 years, she is the mother of three. Her libido vanished on the heels of a death in the family several years ago, when she was in her early forties and married just 12 years.

"I think the problem was multifaceted, multicaused," she says today, "but it seemed to stem from taking antidepressants. I had started taking Zoloft in early '94 and noticed the change in libido pretty quick, but I had undergone such a horrible period of depression after my mother's death and I was going through infertility issues, things like that. But I was feeling so much better because of the medication that I wanted to stick with it even though the loss of libido made me very sad. That was the cause of stress in and of itself.

"At first, I had so many other issues going on that it wasn't my primary concern. But after a year went by, it became more of a concern because I'd been married for 16 years and had always had a wonderful physical relationship with my husband."

According to Dr. Simon, Lauren's reaction to the drug was not unusual. "We don't understand exactly why or how the SSRI/antidepressants (serotonin reuptake inhibitor antidepressants) cause this," he said, "but the link is there even if we cannot say that the antidepressant drug itself lowers the testosterone level. It is also difficult to know whether the sexual problems are related to the depression itself or to the medication treatment."

Lauren complained to her psychiatrist and they tried other drugs to cut down on the sexual side effects. But nothing worked. "I tried going off the Zoloft with really disastrous results as far as the onset of depression," she said. "Then I tried a variety of antidepressants none of which worked as far as treating the depression, so I went back on Zoloft after a couple of months—without a whole lot of relief from the loss of libido."

Next she approached her gynecologist. "A friend had told me about seeing something about a testosterone cream being available to women at this point. So I talked to my doctor but she didn't like the idea of that at all. She said, 'Oh it can have awful side effects on women.' And really discouraged me.

"A year later I talked to her again and said I was still having this problem. Apparently, during that year she had heard some better things. Since it wasn't her area of expertise, she referred me to Dr. Simon. Finally, I was able to get some relief."

Lauren's difficulty in getting current medical advice on how to deal with her loss of libido is not unusual. Most of the women who reach Dr. Simon's office have spent several years and been through two or more physicians in their search for help. For those women not living on the east coast—most of Dr. Simon's patients live in major cities up and down the eastern seaboard—the difficulty is even greater. In Chapter Eight, we will recommend ways to find gynecologists who have the endocrinology background necessary to help a woman determine if testosterone is a healthy option for her.

Lauren was able to meet with Dr. Simon in the spring of 1998— four years after her mother's death and the onset of her depression and consequent loss of libido. "I had a consultation and he suggested testosterone injections because I was not yet menopausal. First, however, he tested my testosterone level. Even now, he has me take blood tests every four or five months to determine the level. But after the first blood work, he said that my testosterone levels were very, very low, extraordinarily low, and he was surprised that I had any kind of sex life at all. I told him that prior to this dropoff in 1994 that I certainly *had* had what I considered to be a pretty good sex life. So he prescribed a low dose of testosterone and we did that for two or three months. I noticed a little bit of a change for a short period of time, but it didn't last very long, maybe a week and a half. And it wasn't anything spectacular. No major difference."

Now it was June. On a Tuesday, Dr. Simon upped her dose.

"I'll never forget what happened next," says Lauren with a wide grin. "Two days later I left on a long road trip with my kids, without my husband, to visit some relatives. I was in the car—this was two and a half days after the injection—I was listening to Dylan singing 'Layla' on the radio when all of a sudden"—she laughs—"it hit me like a ton of bricks! And of course it was terrible timing because I didn't see my husband for a week and a half. But when I got home . . .

"Maybe it was the song that triggered something, but I just went crazy. I remember talking to my husband on the phone every day and telling him how much I couldn't wait to see him.

"And it's just been so fantastic! I thought I had a great sex life before, but I really didn't. I think about this a lot because it has made a huge difference in our marriage.

"Before, when my libido was so low, I tried to explain why that was but I don't think my husband really understood. He took it personally and was very frustrated by it. I did a lot of pretending at that time because I wanted the closeness, but I have to say that when it came to sex I was turned off to the point of being revolted. That's how bad it was. It really was. I tried to hide that, and not always successfully. I mean, we were having sex less than once a week and if it had been up to me—it would have been never."

Lauren's words are reminiscent of the feelings that Sheila had when Ben first moved back into the bedroom. But the revulsion is gone, replaced with a healthy, happy frequency of sexual relations averaging three times a week or more. Aside from her enhanced libido, Lauren has experienced two other side effects. One is an increase in facial hair, confined to her chin, which she bleaches. "It's something I'm willing to put up with." The other is an increase in energy.

"My regret," says Lauren, "is that I didn't do this sooner and I really don't care if taking testosterone is natural or unnatural—I just love it. Frankly, I can't get enough, which makes my husband happy.

"What I've learned through this is that when we're happy in bed, we're happy outside of bed and the more often we're happy—the better we are everywhere. I love my husband. I want to live the rest of my life this way and I hope that I can."

Finally . . . Defining Female Sexual Response and Female Sexual Disorders

No doubt you're wondering why, if libido—and the intimacy it generates—is so important to us, why isn't it easier to fix it when things go awry?

Unfortunately, there have been no accurate models of what a healthy, normal female sexual response *is*, much less what it is *not*.

Without such guidelines in place, physicians have found it difficult to help women who complain of a loss of libido or other sexual disorders. Furthermore, to date the FDA has never clearly defined "female sexual dysfunction" (FSD) as a treatable condition. This means pharmaceutical companies, such as those who manufacture testosterone, have not been able to state that their drugs can be used to treat loss of libido or any other sexual disorder. Bottom line: *No legally defined condition means no legally approved treatment.*

However, this conundrum is about to come to a screeching halt. The FDA has been studying the medical evidence that FSD does indeed exist and they will be providing their final guidelines very soon, hopefully before this book is published. When they do, treatment will be available. After all, the FDA certainly recognizes *male* sexual dysfunction—hence we have the overwhelming success known as Viagra.

In the meantime, Dr. Rosemary Basson of Vancouver, B.C., Canada, as a followup to an international panel discussion on female sexual dysfunction (FSD), has written a paper describing a model for defining FSD in a way that further clarifies the guidelines being recommended to our FDA and other international health agencies.

Dr. Basson attended the international panel, which consisted of 19 experts in female sexual dysfunction drawn from Canada, Denmark, Italy, the Netherlands and the United States. Their backgrounds included endocrinology, family medicine, gynecology, nursing, pharmacology, physiology, psychiatry, psychology, rehabilitation medicine and urology. Each of the panelists is actively involved in research or treatment of female sexual disorders.

While the International Consensus Development Conference drew up new definitions and classifications of women's sexual response, Dr. Basson's paper extended those definitions. A review of the Consensus definitions and Dr. Basson's recommendations in her followup paper, "The Female Sexual Response: A Different

Model," are very illuminating. Whether or not these specific words are formally accepted by government agencies, I think you will find the descriptions to be of great value in helping you determine if you are having a problem with low libido or another sexual disorder. They certainly provide a vocabulary for describing your situation to your partner or your physician. And, throughout, the definitions underscore how closely our sexual needs are tied to our desire for intimacy, to our entire sense of self.

Dr. Basson makes this point early in her paper as she states that medical experts need to recognize that a woman's sexual response originates not from a need for physical sexual arousal but—very likely and more often—from her need for intimacy. As you have seen earlier in this chapter, our need for intimacy has much more to do with our entire sense of self than just who we are below the waist. Thus you may find it no surprise that Dr. Basson goes on to say that earlier medical studies of women's sexuality tended to ignore the concept that sexual satisfaction is a result of intangibles such as "trust, intimacy, the ability to be vulnerable, respect, communication, affection and pleasure from sensual touching." Sociologists, however, have long recognized this.

She goes on to say, too, that at the beginning of a new relationship a woman may have a *spontaneous* urge for sex. Basson has observed that this changes in a longer term relationship where she is more likely to be *responsive* to sexual cues from her partner. For example, she may sense an opportunity for sexual relations, pick up on her partner's interest and readiness, or simply need what flows from sex—the closeness that may result. Either impetus needs to be recognized as perfectly normal.

And she does something else in her paper, which is very pertinent to this book. While she remarks that any attempt to "stage" the female sexual response "is artificial," she does provide a tangible illustration of dysfunction: "the abrupt loss of ovarian androgen."

Such women, writes Dr. Basson, experience these symptoms: "loss of sexual thoughts, dreams and fantasies . . . a loss of the need to self-stimulate and may also lead to the inability to respond to [sexual] cues and triggers that would have elicited sexual desire . . . reduced spontaneous and responsive desire . . . associated lack of response of genital and nongenital areas . . . delay in and reduction of the intensity of orgasm." She feels that this condition reflects all the elements needed to accurately define female sexual disorders in their variety. Is this not the experience many of us have after menopause?

While this may sound like bad news for those of us with an androgen deficiency, that is hardly the case. It is enlightening even as it frees us to seek help. If experts like Dr. Basson can prove it, if authorities will accept that proof, then physicians will listen and help.

And while Dr. Basson's statements may seem obvious to women, they are less so to governing authorities, many of whom have traditionally been male and have judged women by male standards. But in contrast to women, men's sexual function and dysfunction has been more easily observed: difficulty having an erection is obvious. Also, women have less of a need to be sexual just to relieve sexual tension. These are just a few of the differences. Thus the delay in defining female sexual dysfunction has stemmed from too many experts trying to fit women into patterns set by men. Luckily, this is changing.

Recognizing a New Criterion: "Causes Personal Distress"

The current crucial view of a woman's sexual response that emerged from the Consensus panel and Dr. Basson's work included the following concept.

At last it is recognized that a woman can be moved to be sexual by the *expectation of increased intimacy*—as opposed to a strong drive for sex independent of the context of her relationship or the environment around her. This recognition is important because it helps you define whether or not you are having a problem with your libido—within the context of your own needs. You should not be held to another woman's standard. For example, no doctor should ever say that just because you have an orgasm once a month, you're fine. Or that not having an orgasm every time you make love means you are not fine. In other words, you choose the guidelines that determine if you are experiencing low libido or any other type of FSD, and these guidelines should be based on *how you used to feel and how your body used to respond* when you were happy with your sexual self. The words that define this key concept will recur in each of the following descriptions and they are: *"causes personal distress."* For now and forever, remember that phrase.

Now, at the risk of getting too technical, Dr. Simon and I would like to include the exact wording of the new definitions of FSD, drawing from Dr. Basson's paper and from an abstract published following an International Consensus Development Conference.

Not only do these show the issues surrounding female sexual dysfunction, but they demonstrate how redefining the traditional four categories of female sexual response disorders will make medical treatment more accessible.

First, regarding sexual desire and hypoactive (*hypo-* means "less than normal") sexual desire disorder (HSDD), there are two suggestions. The 1998 Consensus panel wrote: "The persistent or recurrent deficiency (or absence) of sexual fantasies, thoughts and/or desire for, or receptivity to, sexual activity, which causes personal distress."

Dr. Basson would like to see this reworded slightly to further clarify the condition. Her suggestion is: "HSDD is the persistent or recurrent deficiency (or absence) of sexual fantasies, thoughts, desire for sexual activity (alone or with partner), *and inability to respond to sexual cues that would be expected to trigger responsive sexual desire*. These symptoms need to be causing personal distress." That phrase, "causing personal distress" is what can prompt you to say to your doctor: "It used to be that kissing and sex play with my husband would trigger sexual interest from me— but I don't feel that way anymore. I'm not interested. I find this confusing and upsetting."

Second, regarding sexual arousal and female sexual arousal disorder (FSAD), the panel noted that many factors confuse the issue. One of these is the simple fact that some areas of a woman's body that are involved in a sexual response are hidden from view; another is that women vary in their awareness of a "marker" such as lubrication. Also, there are many women with healthy sexual desire who may become estrogen-deficient and complain of dryness or pain during intercourse yet they do not lack a sense of sexual arousal.

Dr. Basson agrees with the 1998 Concensus definition for FSAD, which states, "The persistent or recurrent inability to attain or to maintain sufficient sexual excitement causing personal distress. It may be expressed as a lack of subjective excitement or a lack of genital lubrication/swelling (or other somatic responses)." She points out that such a description allows for a woman to be lubricated but lacking "mental excitement" to be diagnosed with FASD—this recognizes the link between our psychology and our biology. It means you can say to your doctor: "My head is willing but my body isn't" or "My heart is willing but my head and body just don't cooperate."

Third, regarding orgasm and female orgasmic disorder (FOD), the 1998 Consensus definition states "orgasmic disorder is the persistent or recurrent difficulty, delay in, or absence of attaining orgasm following sufficient sexual stimulation and arousal and causes personal distress." Basson prefers this definition as it recognizes that if a woman's experience of having or not having an orgasm is not distressing to her, she does not have a dysfunction.

As an aside in her paper, she makes two observations that I found very interesting. First, she notes that clinical experience has shown that contrary to the Masters and Johnson model of a woman achieving orgasmic release, each of us may experience a variety of orgasms. Masters and Johnson noted that women can have more than one "peak" but Basson—after listening to so many women telling their stories—confirmed that these can be "multiple, extended, vary according to circumstance and occasion, and, at times, unnecessary." You may experience one type while masturbating, another as a result of direct stimulation to the vulva and yet another during sexual intercourse. You may experience a breathtaking "peak" in one encounter or a soft, pleasurable "shudder" in another. As Dr. Basson explains, "Orgasmic release is extremely variable and not essential for sexual satisfaction for women." The point is that the new definition allows for every woman to define her personal experience. She is dysfunctional only if she feels her responses are "causing personal distress."

Second, referring back to the example of a woman with an androgen deficiency (note: this could be a low level of testosterone), Basson describes such a woman as ". . . experiencing some arousal . . . some genital tension felt . . . sometimes there is a rather unexpected peak and release but more often they describe their orgasm as 'a little blip on the screen.' " Because this description is surfacing again and again among postmenopausal women, the possibility of prescribing a pharmaceutical to relieve the symptom is becoming more and more likely.

Research into the female orgasm continues but these definitions are proving very helpful. Already, clinical research is showing that women on certain serotonin reuptake inhibitors (SSRIs) or antidepressants and women whose alcohol intake is of a certain level are better able to describe their feelings of female orgasmic disorder now that they have a broader palette by which to describe their past patterns of orgasmic responses.

And, finally, a new category has been acknowledged: sexual pain disorder. This includes recurrent or persistent genital pain associated with sexual intercourse and with noncoital sexual stimulation.

And so the experts are redefining the many causes and multiple dimensions of women's sexual dysfunction patterns. The new female model differs significantly from a man's physiology as the interplay of biological, psychological and interpersonal elements are better recognized.

Now that research results show that up to 40 percent of American women experience some degree of sexual dysfunction—fully a third of American adult women report a lack of sexual interest and nearly a fourth say they do not experience orgasm—the need for relief is underscored. The role hormones can play, particularly testosterone, is evident. A woman's ability to gain access to testosterone through her physician is also necessary. This means it is time for definitive FDA guidelines so that treatments can be developed.

The Testosterone Experience: Exactly What Happens If I Use It?

Four

Eve and Kate:
Naturally Menopausal

E ve is 52 years old. Tiny in stature and armed with piercing
black eyes, she is the architect of one of the nation's most
successful telecommunications companies. The mother of two
young women in their twenties, she recently married for the second
time. When asked about her sense of herself as a sexual being
throughout her life, Eve is quick to say she has always felt confident.

"Early in my high school years, I found myself very attracted
to guys and to the extent that I experimented sexually I enjoyed
it and looked forward to it and sought it. But there were just so
many 'shoulds' and 'shouldn'ts' about sex in those days that I
don't think I gave full expression to my sexual feelings until I was
married."

She married at 22 and soon discovered a discrepancy between

herself and her partner. "I thoroughly enjoyed the sex," said Eve, "and I would say I had a very strong libido. Interestingly enough, my first husband did not. And I would also say that I was probably more the aggressor. He just did not have a particularly strong sex drive."

Did this have an effect on intimacy in the marriage?

"A tremendous effect," said Eve. "Not only a feeling of loss of something missing, but it dampened the sense of fun and enjoyment in the marriage. And as time went on—we were married nearly twenty years—I felt rejected. That grew into anger. I don't think that can be seen in isolation because there were other factors affecting our marriage as well. But absolutely, I think that early on the intimacy was severely compromised and then it became an even larger part of the scenario that led to our divorce."

Six months after formally separating from her husband, Eve met a new man. She also rediscovered a part of herself. "I had been celibate for at least the last year that I was in the marriage and maybe longer, but definitely the last year.

"So when I met Marty, it was a second sexual awakening. It was almost like the first time I had sex as a kid where it was so explosive and so amazing. Except add to that the fact that Marty was tremendously romantic and sexual and inventive. We just had so much fun."

And so she married for the second time. Shortly after her marriage, at age 43, she was stunned to find herself going through menopause.

"Now when I think back," said Eve, "I can see I had early symptoms—feeling bloated, feeling uncomfortable. At first it didn't have an effect on my sexuality and our sexual relations continued on a very active level because we have a strong physical attraction to one another. But then, as I got closer to menopause, I started to have other physical manifestations—the hot flashes and the mood swings, all of which indicated that my estrogen and testosterone levels were decreasing.

"But at the same time the doctor I had been seeing ignored my complaints so I did not get any hormone replacement therapy. Nothing. He refused to even do a blood test.

"Then my libido definitely decreased. Plus the fact that I was just physically so miserable. I wasn't sleeping, I had these mood swings, everything.

"During a break at work, I decided to go to the Canyon Ranch Spa where I had my blood tested. That doctor told me my estrogen level was very low and gave me a prescription for estrogen. What happened next was very interesting. Even though she told me not to expect a change for a while, I'm telling you that the very first pill that I put in my mouth, within probably a day I was starting to feel better.

"However, the libido did not come back. The mood swings left, the hot flashes left, the bloating diminished, all of the other symptoms. But the libido did not return."

Now, even though she felt much better physically, Eve remained acutely aware of a major change.

"My husband and I certainly were still sexual, but it wasn't like I was totally eager. It was more like reliving the memory. For old times' sake more than anything. And yet I was still, in every way, just so mad about him and attracted to him—but I just didn't feel like having sex. And he would be the aggressor more often where before it was more even between us. Also, earlier, when he was the aggressor, I was totally cool with it. But now, it was like 'Uh, okay.' I just wasn't that excited about it."

The low libido confused Eve—along with something else, something less tangible.

"I was puzzled. What was wrong? Here I was married to a guy I adored. I had a fabulous job and I was highly successful in that job. My kids were finishing college. I had a great apartment. For the first time probably ever in my adult life I had no money worries. Everything was great. And yet I had this free-floating anxiety. I just had this sense of dread that something terrible was going to happen, something was not right.

"So that summer I made an appointment to see my shrink. I told him, 'I'm miserable and I don't know why.' I went over every physical and emotional detail, but just like my first doctor at no time did he say, 'you know, these are common symptoms of menopause. Let's look at your hormone replacement therapy.' He never brought that up.

"Instead, we did a whole summer of psychotherapy and, guess what? We couldn't find anything. There was nothing to cause the free-floating anxiety that I was feeling.

"Early that fall, thank goodness, I had dinner with a friend who told me about the estrogen and testosterone she was taking—she was taking it specifically for low libido. While she was talking, I thought 'Oh my gosh, that is exactly what I'm feeling.' So I went home and I called my doctor, only this time I had picked a new ob/gyn, a woman who specializes in menopause. She's about my age. She's terrific. She's handled every other aspect of this whole menopause adventure expertly. So I called her and said I have free-floating anxiety and loss of libido and I was talking to someone who told me about her experience with the testosterone replacement and I thought maybe I should try it.

"She said, 'Oh no, I don't recommend it.' She said, 'Long-term we don't know what the effects of it are, with cancer, with this, with that, and I don't recommend it.' So I said, 'Okay,' and I ended the conversation. Then I called her back shortly after and said, 'I want to go on it. I'm willing to take the risk. I really need to see if this addresses these symptoms.'

"And sure enough, she put me on Estratest and the free-floating anxiety disappeared. It was like I never thought about it again. It totally disappeared without my even noticing it. And my libido is certainly improved, although I would not say that it is absolutely where it used to be. I have asked my doctor if I can increase my dosage but she has said, 'No, no, no, you're at exactly the levels that are safe.'

Eve has been taking Estratest for five years. How does she feel about it today?

"It's a life saver," she says by phone from her office in Los Angeles. "I have to be functioning at a very high level. I have eighty million dollars in revenue riding on my shoulders for my company. And I can't be dealing with this free-floating anxiety stuff, and I can't be dealing with a marriage that's coming apart because I don't want to have sex with my husband. I can't be dealing with those things. I have to be operating at a high level, top form. So I need this. It's funny when I say I'm willing to take the risk. Of course, I don't want to end up with cancer. And if I do, I'm sure I'll look back and say, 'Was it worth it?'

"And I don't know exactly what the answer will be—but right now, my answer is 'Yes. Without question—yes.' "

*   *   *

Fifty-six-year-old Kate is single and has always been single. She is very independent and spirited and has run her own international business for more than twenty years. With a rounded, lush figure and an open Irish face complemented with a smokey, musical voice, she looks much younger than her age.

Though she has chosen to remain single, Kate has had several long-term, satisfying relationships with men. Sex and intimacy have always been important in her life. So when menopause complicated that, her life grew complicated, too.

"I began to feel really, really, really sexy when I was 15," recalls Kate. "I fell madly in love with a boy who was 21. Then, again when I was in college, I fell in love over summer vacation. I've had some wonderful guys in my life."

One reason Kate may never have married was the nature of her business: She moved around the country quite frequently over the years. Still, not being married did not mean she couldn't enjoy sex. "I went through my 30s being fairly sexually active," she said. "During those years I lived in San Francisco, then went back to New York, and ultimately to the southeastern seaboard in '78. And I was fairly sexually active through all of that time."

Menopause entered Kate's life when she turned 40. "And I'm still in it," she says today. "I'm 56 years old and I'm still dealing with symptoms. Today I take Estratest but I couldn't find the right hormone therapy until two years ago. So I went for 14 years being shuttled around and shunted back and forth on different medications, then years with no medication and slightly thinning bones and mood swings—and loss of libido.

"For the longest time I felt like this dried up little raisin of a woman. And I thought that sex was over for the rest of my life, that there would be no more. I remember those years—from 1990 to '96. I had about five years of abstinence because I wasn't interested and it hurt."

Kate's menopause started early with irregular periods. "I would miss one every three or four months," she said. "I was pretty sexually active at the time so I kept thinking I was pregnant and running off to clinics and then running off and buying the home pregnancy tests and being in a panic. That was in 1985.

"In 1987, when I was about 44, I started taking estrogen and it made me feel very ill. The libido was gone, of course, but that may have been confused with everything else physical that was wrong. I was nauseous all the time. Really nauseous. So I stopped taking the estrogen. That didn't help the other symptoms like vaginal dryness and pain."

Kate's experience with the estrogen drugs available in the late '80s shows just how important it is for a woman to find exactly the right combination for her body's chemistry.

"I started taking estrogen again—and I started feeling lousy again but I didn't know for sure that it was the estrogen. So I started going to internists and gastroenterologists to find out why I was so bloated all the time, why I felt like I had a beach ball in my stomach. That was the spring of '87 and I'd met a wonderful man that February but we never had sex because I didn't feel like I could, it hurt so much. I was worried. I was horrified. I felt embarrassed. I felt like I was shrinking up. And I didn't know that all of these were symptoms of menopause."

Kate refused to give up: "I tried different types of estrogen. I went to yet another gastroenterologist in South Carolina, had all those tests for the second or third time in like a year, and then I had a colonoscopy and they found polyps, so I thought maybe that was why I was sick. But I didn't get to feeling any better afterwards so now I was more convinced the problem was the estrogen.

"And like everybody in those days, I was taking estrogen for a certain number of days and progesterone for a certain number. My doctor at the time insisted it wasn't the estrogen causing me to feel bad but I told him the only time in the month when I felt good was the five days at the end when I was not taking estrogen. They wouldn't believe me. I could not persuade any gynecologist that the estrogen could possibly be doing this to me."

Now Kate did give up—on estrogen. "I finally took myself off of it in 1989 because I decided that I knew my body better than my doctors, and I stopped taking it. And I didn't take it again, really, until I found Dr. Simon in December of 1997.

"I had moved again so I had a new ob-gyn. This was around 1993 and my health was still not great. I had no energy, no libido, no appetite, no anything. My new doctor kept me off estrogen but he started me on testosterone—first injections, then pellets. That was good but not great. It gave me more energy and improved my libido, but it didn't help the vaginal dryness very much. Then my doctor retired and Dr. Simon was recommended to me."

Under Dr. Simon's care, Kate's hormone replacement therapy was significantly changed with very positive results. Key to this was Simon's expertise in choosing a type of estrogen that, paired with testosterone, would work for Kate's particular body chemistry.

"The first time I saw him, he said, 'I can't let you keep doing testosterone without estrogen,' " recalls Kate. " 'But I get so sick,' I told him, and he said, 'I promise you this will not make you sick. I promise you.' And it did work! It's been a little over three years now and I've been really fine ever since."

And what is the magic combination that works for Kate?

"I have two pellets inserted under the skin every five or six months: one estrogen and one testosterone. And I take diuretics along with potassium to counteract any damage that could be done by the diuretic."

"Pellets are the answer for someone like Kate," says Dr. Simon, "because they act in a way that allows the hormones to bypass the liver and go straight into the bloodstream. This significantly reduces the opportunity for a reaction to the estrogen."

Kate could not be more enthusiastic over the difference this regimen has made. "I can physically feel a major difference," she said, "when my testosterone is running out, my energy level goes way down. Dr. Simon tests my blood every time before I get new pellets so we can see how low it is. But I don't need to see the test, I can feel it."

Kate is quite happy with the state of her health today, saying, "I am right where I want to be. I got my libido and my energy back with the testosterone and the estrogen relieved the vaginal dryness. And more good news—my cholesterol level has dropped from about 337 to about 218. And my diet is much better because I don't put weight on like before. Now, if I don't go overboard, I can eat almost anything.

"But, really, it was more than just that. I became interested in life again, interested in men and sex and food and music. The testosterone really gave me my life back."

To see Kate today—her eyes happy, her skin lovely under the soft waves of her strawberry blonde hair—you can see how good she feels. No blood test needed for that!

How long does she plan to keep taking the combination of estrogen and testosterone?

"Probably till the day I die. After all, the only side effect I have is some extra facial hair from time to time. Some I pluck and some I trim off with nail scissors. So I may have a lot more facial hair than I did, but understand that I've been on this for a very long time now, nearly six years. It's definitely worth it."

Would she recommend this to others?

"Very much so. I've recently become very aware of how many marriages disintegrate when a woman reaches menopause. I see it in my friends who have had happy marriages. I've talked to the husbands about it because I can relate. I didn't want to have sex for a good seven or eight years when I was feeling so bad.

"These guys are telling me their wives are like that—not interested in them anymore. As a result, the guys go through very lonely times. It's not just the sex—but the sex is the glue, the sex leads to touching and cuddling. You know," Kate shakes her head, "that's what all the guys say, the affection—the hand holding, the hugs—it's disappeared. And the men start wondering if it's their problem. It's very sad.

"So I listen and sympathize and make some suggestions and try to explain what the wives are going through. But, yes, I do recommend this for other women. Menopause is really bad for many of us, but it sure as hell is bad for the people who love us, too."

The Testosterone Experience: Reviewing the Pros and Cons for the Naturally Menopausal Women Interviewed

Pros: Restored libido, increased energy, mood enhancement with a marked decrease in depression and free-floating anxiety, lower cholesterol and less body fat.

It should be noted that not all women experience depression and free-floating anxiety with menopause. For example, I didn't. What I did notice—once I had begun to take testosterone—was an "evening out" of my moods and a consistent sense of well-being.

Cons: A modest increase in facial and other hair growth—but no one has claimed this condition is unmanageable. Some mild acne, which disappeared after a few months.

Warning: Any consideration of testosterone for use by a naturally menopausal woman should be done *only under the care of a physician* who is prepared to calibrate the exact amount and frequency of use for each woman's body chemistry—and monitor this use on a regular basis. In Chapter Seven we will describe a transdermal testosterone patch, applied to the skin, that will reach the market sometime in the next few years. It offers the advantage of enhancing testosterone levels without affecting estrogen, bypassing the liver and eliminating many negative side effects.

Five

Marcy and Hope:
Surgically Menopausal

V ivacious, forthright Marcy is 53 years old. Recently retired from a very successful career as an industrial engineer, she now lives in Chicago with her second husband.

As we sit chatting in a bistro on a sunny spring day, Marcy glows. Her thick auburn hair is tied back. Her wide-spaced dark eyes are warm and humorous as she talks of the sabotage her hormones wreaked on her first marriage—and the second chance at life that a combination of estrogen and testosterone have made possible . . . *after thirty years.*

To see her, so trim and elegant, to listen to her honey-toned voice, you would never suspect the degree to which she has been betrayed by her body. It started early, like it does for so many of the more than 30 million women in the United States who are surgically menopausal.

"When I was 16, I had a cyst removed from my ovary," said Marcy. "At the same time they removed half of one ovary and two-thirds of the other. Two years later I had more cysts removed. But I hung in there, got married at 22 and had twins. I was very fortunate. Not only was I able to have children, but they turned out to be healthy and quite normal.

"I, however, was not normal. The following year I had exploratory surgery and my doctor recommended a hysterectomy. So at age 24 I had twins and no female system and that was only the beginning. I was immediately put on estrogen and at age 30 I had a mild stroke.

"The doctors didn't know *why* I had this stroke, but after many tests and neurological exams they decided that I had had too much estrogen. So they took me off hormones altogether. I was 32 years old when I went through an early menopause."

How do you cope with such a major physical change when you are still a young woman, a woman who should be sexually active, who may have wanted more children?

"You become a workaholic," said Marcy. "Even though I was feeling pretty rotten with hot flashes and all, my career was taking off. So I propelled myself into my work, focussing on that and the care of my children. My husband was an engineer, too, which meant we were both working extremely hard.

"Then, after the stroke, I went through more changes. Since I wasn't on estrogen any longer, my female system dried up. Because I had no libido, I didn't feel like having sex. I had incredible energy but it was directed elsewhere. The end result was no physical relationship with my husband. We kept it together for a while, but by the time I was 44, we were getting a divorce."

Would she blame the divorce on her surgery and early meno-pause?

"Absolutely. It was *the* problem. We were dear friends and close business associates and we had everything going for us, but there was just no intimacy. None at all.

"It wasn't like I didn't try," said Marcy, echoing the words of many of the women interviewed for this book who sought out doctor after doctor trying to solve this problem. "By the time we separated, I had been through complete workups with four differ-ent neurologists at all the best hospitals—major players.

"But they all said the same thing: 'You may not take oral es-trogen at all. Ever again.' So I didn't take it even though, by then, I was in terrible shape. My vaginal area was so dry that I had blisters and sores. I couldn't even wear slacks. I mean, my female system was a mess. And mentally, I felt like a eunuch."

This drove Marcy even further into her career—and her hus-band into the arms of another woman.

"I think what happened was he felt so badly for me because I had these visible sores—that he retreated. Yes, we would hold hands and, yes, we seemed close friends, but we had not had sex-ual relations for seven, maybe eight years," recalls Marcy. "He became impotent with me. And I think it forced him to reexamine himself, what he wanted . . . needed . . . out of life.

"Again, it's not like we didn't try. We went through heavy doses of therapy. But he found somebody else." She pauses. "It was classic: my best friend. When it happened, I was indignant and unhappy and all that, but looking back, I don't blame him. The poor guy. It was bad for both of us because of my situation and, at that time, no one could offer any alternative."

What about the insistence of some women that a sexual relationship isn't always necessary to a good marriage?

"But sex is such a rich part of life," counters Marcy. "We weren't ignoring that. Our therapists were offering sexual support and it did help a little bit. But the friendship between the two of us was all we really had. The time came when we realized that there was not going to be any more than that—and that wasn't enough for the man to whom I was married.

"So we separated and went our own ways. And I felt tremendous guilt, that it was *I* who broke up the marriage."

Not long after her divorce, Marcy got an unexpected phone call. "An estrogen *patch* had come out. My doctor called and said, 'There's a new estrogen delivery system on the market and I would like to hold your hand and get you through this.' "

Estrogen? For a woman who had experienced a mild stroke when taking it earlier?

"At first, I balked," said Marcy. "I didn't need another stroke. But he said, 'Marcy, I know there's hypersensitivity. I know we've tried all these creams and baths and they haven't worked. Still, I'm very concerned about infection in the vaginal area. We'll start slow, we'll start by cutting the patch into eighths.' " He also explained that the patch would deliver the estrogen directly to her bloodstream, bypassing the liver and limiting the likelihood of side effects.

"That's what we did and I was okay. Then, over the next six months, we eased up the dosage. My doctor monitored every step with blood tests, blood pressure exams, and checks of my arteries to make sure that everything was flowing just right. It worked!

"Within a year, my dryness was gone, the blisters had disappeared and I had begun to feel pretty good. The only problem was I had started to put on weight. I'm 5'5" and my weight had been steady at around 140 pounds, which worked for me. I looked pretty thin and I could wear a size 8 or 10. But by this time I was 47 years old so I assumed some weight gain was natural for my age. I didn't pay too much attention at first."

Three years later, just as she turned fifty, life took an interesting turn for Marcy. She gave a lecture one evening and a fellow engineer lingered to chat. Soon afterward, he invited her to dinner at his home. To her great surprise, the relationship bloomed.

"My divorce had been so traumatic that I wasn't expecting to meet anyone. After all, I hadn't had sexual relations with my first husband for so many years, I didn't know if I could even *have* a physical partner—or *want* to. Then I met this man and I was stunned at my response to him."

Stunned and confused.

"It started that first night that we had dinner together. I took one look at the plates he had set out on his dining room table and I was spooked: *We have the same china*. This is not everyday china. It is a very ornate, very expensive pattern that you don't see often."

Marcy laughs, remembering how she felt. "I was so shaken, I had to excuse myself. 'Would you mind if I take a five-minute breather here?' I said. 'I need to sit down, I'm not feeling real well.' So I went into his family room and started looking at his CDs. It so happens I had just spent two summers in Spain and had fallen in love with classical Spanish music—*he had the same CDs*! That was it. I knew right away something special was happening.

"Even though we saw each other a lot over the next few months and were amazed at how much we had in common, when he would try to kiss me, I would push him back. As attracted as I was, I just did not want that kind of a relationship. I was very much against getting married or having a long-term relationship. I did not want to allow myself to be vulnerable. I did not want any of those things again. I guess I didn't think I could function as a woman even if I did want it.

"Then it happened—and the first time he kissed me I thought the world would stop. That's when I knew that he needed to know about me."

Marcy forced herself to tell Philip what she was sure would end the relationship.

" 'Look here, bud,' I said finally, 'there's a big thing I've got to tell you. And I'm truly frightened. I care a lot more for you than I thought I was capable of. I would like to explore it further, but I'm frightened about the physical nature of our relationship.' "

She gave him all the details. His response was unexpected.

"He shared with me that he was diabetic and had physical limitations himself—he can't sustain an erection. We talked about how we could help each other in that regard, explore all this together."

Within weeks, Marcy and Philip had made a decision to resign their high-pressure jobs, get married and travel abroad. This time together led to yet another mutual decision.

"We were so happy," said Marcy. "During those three months I learned to relax, to calm down, to focus on my partner and on my own needs and desires. That trip was a great starting point for our marriage. And we were married probably a week when I said to him, 'I'd really like to find out more about the sexual side of my situation.' He felt the same and said, 'I'm going to find out more about my problem, too.' We agreed that what we had together so far was really great and maybe we could improve on it.

"When we got back, I saw my internist. I had lots of questions for him. When I said I had very low libido and wondered if more estrogen might improve that, he recommended Dr. Simon. His own wife was seeing Dr. Simon, taking testosterone and feeling terrific. And because Dr. Simon is an ob/gyn who specializes in hormone research, my internist felt I should try working with him instead. Also, by now my weight gain had gotten out of control. I had put on twenty pounds and felt like a beach ball. So with ten pounds on each hip, I marched myself into Dr. Simon's office.

"That first visit was frustrating," recalls Marcy. "Dr. Simon started out by telling me not to be surprised if my low libido was caused by depression in which case he would recommend a psychiatrist rather than testosterone. Excuse me? I explained to him in a rather testy way that depression was not very likely, that I had a new partner, that I was deliriously happy in my marriage— which I *was*—and that I was pretty happy with my physical condition, too, except for the weight gain. But he was cautious.

"Fortunately, the results of my blood test proved *me* right: My testosterone levels were nonexistent, even the estrogen was low. After meeting with both my husband and myself, he started me on testosterone injections, keeping the estrogen at the same level. A few months later, we upped the estrogen, even though we had to try four different patches before we found the right one.

"That was eighteen months ago. I continue to have monthly testosterone injections, though the dosage is slightly lower than the level at which I started."

And the results? Marcy is thrilled.

"Talk about libido—I have incredible libido. It has changed me so much. I've lost eight pounds of the 20 and working on it. But more than anything, I have a lot of energy, positive energy. I have this little smile on my face. I always feel content. And I really attribute that to the testosterone.

"Something else that is very interesting is the change in Philip. As I've undergone the testosterone treatment and become more aggressive myself—not demanding, but more aware of my own physical needs—he has changed, too. He realizes that he's been missing out on a lot. He's aware of his own needs. So we have a kind of coming together here.

"We still have times when he can't sustain an erection, but we find alternatives. Our love for each other seems to be on a different plane and when the passion takes over it's like our bodies know where to go, and you know, we resolve it. It's wonderful for me especially because as a young woman, my system was so screwed up that this is all brand-new for me. All brand-new. And I hope it stays this way the rest of my life."

What about side effects?

"I have had a little facial hair and I've gone to waxing," said Marcy. "First I tried bleaching, but I get a facial every month so it is easy to have the waxing. I also went from—and I'm really not exaggerating now—I went from ten hairs in my pubic area to just hair all over. For years after my hysterectomy I had no pubic hair. And now I do. It is amazing. I have to shave my legs again, too.

"But no complaints. I've laughed with my husband any number

of times. I've said, 'I'm so grateful to have pubic hair again.' Makes me feel sexy."

Looking back over the last few years, how does Marcy feel about testosterone and estrogen and the effect these hormones have had on her life?

"You can see the answer by looking at us," said Marcy with an easy smile. "I'm 53 and my husband is 63 with diabetes and high blood pressure—and we enjoy having sex two or three times a week. We're in a constant state of 'newlywed.' It may not always be mad, passionate sex, but there's an intimacy between us that I have never experienced before. Never.

"For too many years, I didn't like my body and, therefore, I didn't like myself and I didn't want anyone near me. For the first time in my life, I like all the things around me and who I am and where I am.

"I only hope that my experience can help someone else. I feel so sorry for a young woman who has to go through a hysterectomy and have no options. I've been there and it's horrible. I have such high regard for Dr. Simon's research and how it will help other women because there's a lot of us out there who have been locked into this for a long, long time.

"Having what I have now, I'm glad that my first marriage didn't make it because it was always a struggle. This is not a struggle. This is so easy for me. I've been with this man every day since we were married two years ago. We've not spent one night apart. We may bump against each other once in a while but the bumps are not even big bumps. It's kind of like he raises his voice, I raise mine, and that's the end of the story. Not that we're hiding anything but we have a very basic understanding of one another, a wonderful kind of peace together."

Hope experienced a surgical menopause much later in life than did Marcy. That surgery plus others proved that she is a woman true to her name. When it comes to maintaining her femininity, this woman has been through a series of physical and emotional losses that appeared to leave her, for a time, with nothing but hope.

At age 49, the research consultant may appear robustly healthy, a vision in a peach sweater that accents the glow of her pleasant, freckled face, but Hope is half the woman she once was.

Hope lost her mother to ovarian cancer and two of three aunts, her mother's sisters, to breast cancer. Four years ago she found herself at very serious risk when she tested positive for the BRCA mutation, a gene that further heightens the risk of breast cancer. To save her life and on the advice of her physicians, Hope elected to have multiple surgeries that would remove all risk. Standing by her through the difficult decision, the operations and her recovery has been her husband of 30 years, Alex.

"Not only did I have a surgical menopause," said Hope, "it was really a one–two punch, physically and psychologically. I had been seeing Dr. Simon even before I had the genetic tests. When the results of those tests came in, I decided I wanted to do all the prophylactic surgeries necessary. I had them all done simultaneously—so on the same day I had the ovaries removed, a total hysterectomy, double mastectomy, and some reconstructive surgery.

"I not only went through menopause but you can imagine the body image and other issues, one on top of the other. So that set the theme of my life just as I turned 46.

"Dr. Simon and my other doctors urged me to do some hormone replacement therapy; they emphasized that because I had lowered the risk so dramatically with the surgeries that raising it a slight amount was worth the tradeoff. But I really didn't want to do any hormones because I had gone through all this to minimize my risk. I was very leery of anything that might increase it.

"Finally, I did do six weeks of Premarin immediately following the surgery. Dr. Simon and my ob-gyn said that even if I wasn't going to do it permanently, I should give myself a break while I was recovering and not have to experience the beginning of surgical menopause as well. So I did that, but after six weeks I quit and didn't do any more HRT for a year and a half."

What changed her mind?

"At first, my bones were more the issue than libido. When I saw Dr. Simon a couple of months after the surgery, he did a baseline bone density test. Again, he urged me to take HRT. He wasn't talking libido then, he was talking bone loss. But I said, 'Let's wait and see.'

"A year and a half later, my bones were much worse, my cholesterol had gone up and I had no libido. But at least I was more comfortable with the idea of taking something.

"And by now libido was a major issue for me. I've been married a long time to the same guy. And I still like him. Even if I characterize our sex life as kind of plain vanilla, we were always sexually active. We liked it. It worked for us. It was comfortable. Sex was a part of my life that I had enjoyed and, believe me, I was missing it.

"I *really* missed it by this time," emphasized Hope. "I'd had some libido when I was on Premarin but now I had reached a point where I was totally inert. Like there was zero. Having never been at that point before, I now realized the enormous difference between nothing and a little. Qualitatively I feel like it's really, really different. Not that I'm ready to settle for just a 'little,' but at least you feel like you're a sexual creature even if you don't have as much interest or whatever.

"The change that happened after the surgery was a huge difference for me. I not only missed being able to have a satisfying sex life but a part of me that I'd totally taken for granted had disappeared. It was like something as vital as my sense of smell was gone. My sense of myself as being sexual is so much a part of being me that it doesn't matter if I have a partner or not, if I masturbate or not. Even if I do nothing to actualize my sex life, I still notice a difference if that sense is missing: I'm not me.

"So I went on the HRT with hope that it would help the bones and the cholesterol but absolutely the libido issue. First Dr. Simon and I tried a couple of estrogen drugs but that didn't do much for my libido, which, by the way, I hadn't yet mentioned to him as a concern of mine. Then I heard about testosterone and libido through a discussion group on the Internet.

"And it was right at that time that Dr. Simon raised the issue. This is something I have valued in my relationship with him—he's quite easy to talk with, usually one step ahead."

Now that Hope was talking about libido and her fear of using HRT had eased, Dr. Simon prescribed an oral combination of estrogen and testosterone, Estratest H.S. Encouraged by the initial changes in her body, including the restoration of some libido and the lack of negative side effects, Hope is enthused and open to further improving her libido if possible. Doctor and patient are proceeding carefully.

"Six months after I started taking Estratest, I told Dr. Simon I'd like to do something more. So recently we have added some topical testosterone. The reason for this is the problem with Estratest is if you want to double the testosterone component, you have to double the estrogen, too, because that's the way it's manufactured. Neither Dr. Simon nor I want to increase the estrogen.

"But when I asked about the topical testosterone, he expressed concern about controlling the quantity. This is a problem—you don't know what the strength is. But I'm trying it, applying it to the clitoris and so far I have had no problems. I feel like I'm seeing a slight effect and if I want to continue this, I'll have a blood test to monitor how much I have in my system.

"Meanwhile, I know I'm being awfully conservative," laughs Hope. "Dr. Simon told me to use half of what you would put on a toothbrush. I mean, how much testosterone would *you* put on a toothbrush? I don't know—my 'half a toothbrush' is pretty small, I think." She laughs again. "But we'll see what works eventually."

A question more serious than her "half a toothbrush" dilemma is this: How has Hope's husband reacted to all the changes she has been through these last four years?

Unlike Marcy, whose surgeries occurred in her twenties when her marriage was young, Hope entered the world of surgical menopause blessed with a buffer: a good marriage of thirty years. Has that made a difference?

"The surgery has been a problem for both of us. He really had some difficulty with my body changes. And that came as an enormous surprise because he has always been very accepting of my looks, never asking me to change my hair or dress a certain way or critical if I put on weight.

"But while he was and is very supportive of the concept behind all my surgeries, he had a strong emotional reaction to the changes in me physically, the strangeness. I can understand . . . kind of. Because the reconstruction process took over a year, I looked pretty odd at first. Like I had skin but nothing that visually resembled a nipple.

"And, by the way, that's a whole other thing that is part of my loss of sexual responsiveness. With the breast surgery, some of my much-valued nerve endings were thrown into a Dumpster. I really miss that sensation. And I hadn't thought about that in advance. I guess I figured I would use some other erogenous zone instead, but I miss it a lot more than I ever expected—and testosterone can't restore that.

"So Alex's reaction to this has been difficult for me. I wanted his affirmation to help me feel feminine again, but he wasn't able to give it. He wasn't rejecting but he wasn't comfortable with my body either. But that was earlier before all the reconstruction was finished. I think he has gotten over that and feels okay now. But I haven't totally regained my self-confidence and, emotionally, I keep thinking, 'What if my body changes in another way?' This hasn't been easy adjusting."

How does he feel about her taking testosterone?

"Very supportive. In fact, he went with me to see Dr. Simon. This issue of increasing my risk in order to have some semblance of a sex life is one we are facing together. It's one we could never have imagined dealing with earlier in our marriage and it has forced us into talking so much more, which is probably a good thing.

"Even though there's no way our marriage has been or would be threatened in terms of whether we stopped feeling an incredibly strong bond between us, the lack of sex in our lives—being just buddies, even if the cuddling was still there—that's not enough for us. It may not be that bad, but it is so much less than what we want.

"So, yes, it makes a huge difference that we're able to be sexually intimate again, though I haven't reached the point that I want. I'm still not at the level of interest of initiating sex. I know my husband doesn't want to always be the initiator, so I want to change that.

"But I'm coming along. I'm more responsive from inside as opposed to just agreeing to sex on principle. But I haven't reached a level where my biological underpinnings make me actually *want* to have sex. Before all this happened to me, I had an emotional response level that I still miss. But as Dr. Simon said when we started Estratest, my testosterone levels were profoundly low—so my body is changing. I'm not where I was but I'm trying to get there. You know, when you lose something, you're so much more appreciative of what you've taken for granted all along.

"As long as I can stay safe, I'll continue to increase the testosterone. This is a very valid choice that I am making."

The Testosterone Experience: Reviewing the Pros and Cons for the Surgically Menopausal Women Interviewed

Pros: Restored libido, more responsive to partner's sexual overtures, increased energy, mood enhancement and less body fat.

Other good news is the possible use of estrogen and testosterone by women like Marcy who have a proven sensitivity to these hormones. This should be done, of course, *only under the care of a physician* who is prepared to calibrate the exact amount and frequency of use for each woman's body chemistry—and monitor this use on a regular basis. Please note that the estrogen *patch* has significantly helped alleviate problems. This should be a benefit of the transdermal testosterone patch, which is soon to reach the market and offer similar advantages.

Cons: A modest increase in facial and other hair growth—but, as Marcy said, "no complaints."

Six

Claire and Matt:
The Premenopausal Couple

B ut what if you are a woman who feels you *have* nothing to restore? Or to rephrase the question: What if you don't know what you're missing because you never had it in the first place? And there is no obvious reason for your low libido because menopause is years away. This was the conundrum facing Claire and her husband.

A close look at Claire and Matt's dilemma shows how a low testosterone level can affect a person of any age with disturbing results for a couple. It also clarifies the long-term impact a *change* in the testosterone level can have on the relationship. What is unique to their story is that we can see this impact from both points of view—wife and husband.

*   *   *

Claire is six feet tall. She is a stunning redhead with serene eyes and an open English-Irish face. At 36, she is seven years younger than Matt, her husband of 14 years, who is as friendly, forthright and tall as his wife.

She is taking a break from a career in nursing to be a stay-at-home mom. He is a successful business executive specializing in insurance marketing and sales. Residents of Baltimore and the parents of two children, ages eight and six months, they are deeply committed to one another and to their marriage.

This was not always the case.

Just three years ago, after a decade of quarrels and tears and massive doses of therapy and marriage counseling, the couple was on the verge of divorce. Claire was suicidal.

The core problem, which they learned when it was nearly too late, was not the couple, but Claire. Beautiful, freckle-faced, long-legged Claire's testosterone level was so low it was nearly nonexistent. It was so low that Claire describes her former self as ". . . never interested in having sex. Never. And never had been, either."

I met Claire and Matt for dinner one night in a restaurant not far from the harbor where they keep their new cabin cruiser. Over a leisurely meal, they shared their story with me in hopes that the details of how they stumbled onto testosterone and how it saved their marriage might help another couple avoid the desperation, acute depression and the anger that nearly destroyed their life together.

"Matt was always willing to do what I wanted," said Claire, "and he was always trying to figure out what I might want, but for the first ten years of our marriage I just didn't want to have sex, period. For example, he always made sure I had an orgasm first, but instead of feeling satisfied, I would be thinking 'Okay, I'll have it so he'll be happy and we can get this over with.' "

"That's how sad it was," says Matt.

Claire nods in agreement. To underscore her husband's remark, she adds, "It was really sad that for so long in our life together, I did not enjoy sex. I can look back now and realize that was at the heart of a constant depression I was feeling—we had no closeness, no intimacy whatsoever."

Things are different today. Today she speaks as a woman who has come to understand what it means to *desire* her husband and to *enjoy* an act of sexual intimacy—and its afterglow of warmth and friendship.

But it has been a long road to reach this point as Claire's low libido first surfaced after puberty. Yet all she noticed at the time was what seemed to be a slight difference between herself and her friends in how she felt about boys and sex.

"I was never interested in sex even though my friends talked about it all the time. From puberty on—*I was just not interested. I only lost my virginity because I was a senior and the boy wanted to and I wanted to keep him as a boyfriend. I figured that's what I was supposed to do.

"Looking back, I don't think I ever had sex because I wanted to, it was always because I *had* to. I met Matt when I was nineteen, so I never had a lot of sexual partners. But the few times I was with men, I would have sex only to keep them. I never *wanted* to make love. I knew it was a necessary part of a relationship, but I also knew that my desire was not there. And I never understood what my friends meant when they said they were 'horny.' "

In spite of her lack of interest in sex, Claire *was* interested in guys. "I liked the concept of having a boyfriend," she recalls. So she was certainly open to Matt's attentions when he entered her life.

"When I met Claire, I knew immediately that I wanted to marry her," says Matt with a broad smile directed to his wife. It's obvious he thought she was gorgeous then and thinks so now.

And how did she feel about him nearly seventeen years ago? "I had never met anyone like Matt. I was very flattered that someone who was so articulate, so good-looking, so self-confident, would be interested in me. So, sure, I was happy to get married. Just like I liked the *idea* of having a boyfriend, I liked the *idea* of being someone's wife."

But was she attracted to Matt in any other way?

"I was as sexually attracted as I *could* be, which wasn't much. So it's always been low. Even our wedding night was a trial," she adds. "I had asked Matt if we could abstain from sex for a couple weeks before the wedding so the night would be more special . . ."

"All those weeks without it were fine for Claire," interjects Matt with a laugh.

"They *were*," said Claire, "and on our wedding night I would much rather have just gone to sleep. So I had this problem from the very beginning."

The problem, which began as a lack of desire and a lack of response to Matt's interest in her, escalated to something more serious.

"Matt needed sex," said Claire. "To be sexually intimate with me made him feel wanted and needed. It was validation, proof that he was being a good husband and a good father. That's not what it meant to me. I thought I could show him I loved him in other ways, but for him it was the sex act that was the fulfillment."

Claire's lack of interest resulted in her withholding sex, responding coolly to Matt's advances.

"When he wasn't getting what he thought he needed, he'd get angry, and then I'd get angry. It would just escalate. But the more he wanted me, the more I withdrew."

"That's right," said Matt. "The more she pushed me away, the more I wanted her—like could we do it twice a day?"

"Once every six months made *me* happy," counters Claire.

The more he badgered, the more she withdrew. "I felt attacked, like a cornered animal." Soon nearly every attempt at sex was ending in fights and anger.

"We were in this death spiral," said Matt.

"A vicious circle," adds Claire. "When we first went to counseling, they told me I had 'performance anxiety,' something that men normally have. That was me: I would feel pursued and just shut down because I knew that I wasn't going to get excited like my husband wanted me to. I felt pressure because I knew my husband wanted to please me and that I wasn't going to be able to follow through."

But what confused the issue for Claire and for the professionals that first tried to help the couple was that even though her initial response was lacking—her basic level of desire—her body would react normally during the next stages. She could experience arousal and orgasm.

"Right," she says. "Once we were making love, I would become aroused and orgasmic. That wasn't the problem. The problem was that mentally I just wasn't there. It was like, 'Okay that's nice.'

And I'd end up angry with my husband for wanting to have sex and guilty because I didn't, guilty even when I had an orgasm because *I didn't really enjoy being with him*." The body was willing but the heart held back.

"And he always thought it was his fault." As she speaks, Claire rests her hand on Matt's. "He thought he was doing something wrong and that was why I had no desire for him."

And so the anger and guilt and depression festered, driving them both into depression, encouraging thoughts of divorce.

Though they went into therapy within two years of their marriage, it would be seven years before they would find the right professional help. Even then the therapists would miss the root cause.

Meanwhile, Claire had begun to think that the problem might be on her side of the marital bed. "I talked to friends who also had low libido but that was because of fatigue from work and kids. They were different from me because they could remember when they had *wanted* to have sex.

"I started to feel like I was missing out on a big part of life. I know God put us here and gave us our bodies for pleasure or whatever, and I was, for some reason, unable to do that and I didn't know why. So between talking to my friends and the therapists, I began to feel something was very wrong with *me*."

The confusion and distress mounted. Finally, depressed to the point of feeling suicidal and ready to file for divorce, Claire agreed to one final round of therapy. This time they picked a husband and wife team.

"We saw them first individually and then as a couple," said Matt.

"It was especially helpful that we both gave permission to our counselors to talk amongst themselves," said Claire. "That helps because there are always two sides to a story. I'd see a problem at one extreme and my husband at the other. Our therapists would compare notes and figure out where the median was."

"They were just great at helping us clear away the emotional rubble," said Matt. "At first, they thought Claire's anger was the block to her libido. So we worked on 'family of origin' issues, money problems, our power struggles, everything. We got rid of all the anger, all the noise between us." He pauses, ". . . *but still no libido.*"

"I was extremely frustrated at that point," said Claire, "because things were going along better than ever before during our entire marriage. We were dealing with our anger issues, we were communicating well, everything was going well *but the libido still was not there.*"

Since they were both being treated for depression, they went off those medications to see if that would make a difference; and Claire stopped taking her birth control pills as they are known to block or depress libido in some women. *Still no change.*

Then serendipity struck. Claire happened to tune in to a television show that featured a woman who had taken testosterone to restore her libido. She made an appointment immediately to see her ob-gyn.

She asked to try testosterone. Her physician, who had been a resident in the hospital where Dr. Simon was conducting his early research, recommended that she see Dr. Simon. "You'll really like him," she told Claire. "He's doing studies on testosterone and he is working with women."

The appointment with Dr. Simon changed Claire and Matt's lives.

"First, they took my testosterone levels, which came back amazingly low. Dr. Simon asked me, 'Are you even having regular periods?' The testosterone levels were so low that in theory I shouldn't have been having a normal period. But, even so, I was.

"Then he explained all the potential side effects of taking testosterone and all of the different options—the pill, the gel or the shots. He recommended the shots, so I started taking them. After the first one, he said, 'Don't go home and put pressure on yourself thinking, "Okay—now it's going to happen!" '

"So I said 'Okay, I won't,' but of course I did." Claire and Matt laugh heartily at the memory.

"We sat and looked at each other waiting for this lightbulb to go off, but it took maybe a week or two to take effect. Then I really started noticing a difference."

Claire's voice softens. "For the first time, I *wanted* my husband. I pursued him. And that put a different spin on things because he had been the pursuer for so long—*and now I was pursuing him*. And I was being very . . . I don't know how to say this . . . very *inventive* and kind of crazy. I was all of a sudden more interested in a playful way and more interested in trying other things. And exploring it. And just having a good time with it. And really enjoying and . . . it's like a lightbulb really did go off!"

She pauses again. "Something happened *biochemically*. This was more than what happens when a man is able to have an erection—this really changed my *attitude*.

"I remember at one point I was being very aggressive and Matt told me later—he was laughing when he said it—but he said, 'That kind of scared me but let's try it again.' He wasn't sure how to deal with it, but he was willing to say, 'Wait a minute, I kind of like this.' "

What *was* Matt thinking during that time? As I asked the question, I watched Matt's face in the dim light of the restaurant. Claire was silent, a soft smile on her lips, her eyes shining as she waited for her husband to answer.

"It was hard for me," said Matt, his voice low and deliberate. "Suddenly there was a whole new dynamic to our relationship. Claire was discovering her sexuality for the first time in her life. She had become more aggressive and I found that intimidating at first because this was not the person I knew her to be. I had to adapt and I am not the most adaptive person."

How long did it take him to adjust to this remarkable change in his wife and their relationship?

"About a month," he says, "and it precipitated a change in me, too. Because we were experiencing more intimacy and the frequency was up, I felt less threatened so the need to 'prey' for sex disappeared. I found myself being less insane, less focused on how *much* I was getting. I mean, today"—he laughs—"I'm a whole lot less frenetic about our sex life—I'll go three or four days and not even think about sex!"

For Claire it was a major life change. "Not only was sex not an anxiety issue anymore, but I changed in other ways, too," she adds. "Before I had always been quiet, holding back, especially around Matt's family, who are all very outspoken and opinionated and love to argue politics. Now I'm more aggressive in every part of my life, emotionally and physically. I speak my mind more easily, I have my own opinions and don't hold back. I feel good about myself. I've joined the family!" she exclaims with a big smile.

"Do you think my aggression is a side effect?" she asks.

Maybe—or maybe it is that wonderful sense of confidence and well-being that other women taking testosterone, including myself, have experienced after starting the hormone. But has she experienced any other side effects?

"No," said Claire, "only that sense of feeling more aggressive. My cholesterol has remained very low and I have no problem losing weight." She pauses. "Except the most wonderful thing happened. We were seeing our therapist a few months after starting my shots when Matt suddenly turned and asked me if I would have a baby with him."

"We were overcome," said Matt. "We went from having a divorce to having a child . . ."

To prepare for getting pregnant, Claire went off the testosterone until after the birth of their baby. "And I've only been back on it for four months," she said. "They want you to have three regular cycles before going back on. Meanwhile, Matt and I were like, 'Okay, okay, when can we go back on it?' And we can really see a big difference. As soon as I went back on it, within a couple of days the libido was back again."

It is now three years since Claire started taking testosterone by injection and six months since the birth of their second child. As we sit in the warm glow of the restaurant, Claire and Matt are in a very different place in their marriage than they were when divorce was too real an option.

Has testosterone made a difference beyond the sex?

They are sitting shoulder to shoulder in the booth across from me, leaning comfortably into each other. They answer in overlapping phrases.

"Our sexual relationship is much more tender," offers Matt. "And we are much more emotionally connected versus it being just a physical act. This emotional connection has taken us to a level where I would use the word 'intimacy' to describe what we have—as opposed to 'sex,' and there is a huge difference between the two in my estimation."

Claire expands on his words. "As a couple, we're definitely having more fun. We're much closer, not only sexually but in all other aspects of our lives. We feel much more bonded and happier, much more content.

"Life is so good for us now. We have a new boat and we're out on Chesapeake Bay every weekend with the kids. We're just enjoying each other, our son and our baby—it's wonderful."

A thoughtful pause around the table as I check my notes to see if I have any more questions . . . Matt breaks the silence. "Isn't my wife a special girl? Isn't she a beautiful, lovely person?"

Claire's face glows in the candlelight. "And he is a wonderful man . . . it just takes me aback to remember how I felt four years ago—so sure I wanted a divorce. And here we are today, thanks to therapy and testosterone."

"Nothing worthwhile is ever easy," says Matt.

As I write this book, Claire and Matt are celebrating 15 years of marriage, a marriage as fresh and exciting as if they were newlyweds. And testosterone helped make it happen: the love, the intimacy, the pleasure and the peace.

*　　*　　*

In summary, Dr. Simon has this to say about young women and testosterone: "We don't know how many women in Claire's age range are likely to have a low testosterone level because no research has been done on younger women. We do know that birth control pills can lower libido in some women and many of the antidepressants will have a similar effect, with or without altered testosterone levels. Women with normal spontaneous menstrual cycles almost always have normal levels of testosterone.

"Claire's case also underscores the need, as discussed in Chapter Three, for the new guidelines defining female sexual dysfunction to include two key phrases: first, ' . . . causes personal distress,' and second, 'an inability to respond to sexual cues that would be expected to trigger responsive sexual desire.'

"In the future, a woman who describes symptoms like Claire's—which were the lack of response to her partner's sexual advances coupled with the stress caused in the relationship by her low libido—should be immediately recognized as experiencing some level of female sexual dysfunction.

"She may be someone for whom, under the care of her physician, testosterone may be an option."

The Testosterone Experience: Reviewing the Pros and Cons for the Younger, Premenopausal Woman Interviewed

Pros: Restored and enhanced libido, more responsive to partner's sexual overtures, increased sense of well-being, no increase in cholesterol levels, ease in losing weight.

Cons: A modest increase in facial and other hair growth.

Any consideration of testosterone for use by a younger woman should be done *only under the care of a physician* who is prepared to document the need for this therapy and calibrate the exact amount and frequency of use for each woman's body chemistry—and monitor this use on a regular basis. Please note that a testosterone patch may soon reach the market and offer the advantage of raising testosterone levels while bypassing the liver, thus reducing negative side effects.

The Testosterone Decision: What to Ask For, How to Ask

Seven

Testosterone Options:
The Benefits, the Risks, the Drugs

L ow libido is not the only reason many of us take testosterone. The benefits are many and range from strengthening our bones, increasing our energy levels, enhancing our moods as well as our cognitive functions—from memory to math skills—to even putting the bounce back into our hair.

This chapter is devoted to heightening your awareness of the benefits and risks, the facts and hypotheses. We will also discuss the current and future ways we may be treated with testosterone with an exclusive focus on FDA-approved medications available by prescription only. This will include drugs currently in use as well as those in the research/development/clinical test pipeline. And, finally, we will take a close look at what may prove to be the healthiest option for many women—the testosterone patch.

Please be aware that hormone research is continually changing, and the information in this chapter is a guide to what is current and new, not a medical opinion that is suitable for everyone. Every woman is a unique individual with a unique body chemistry.

Your physician has the role and responsibility of making diagnostic and treatment decisions, discussing them with you, giving you the benefit of his or her medical opinion and devising the hormone replacement therapy most appropriate to your situation. *Do not pursue any hormone replacement therapy unless you are under the care of a physician or other licensed health care provider.*

Testosterone: The Benefits and Risks

As you may have noted in the earlier chapters, testosterone can be taken in several different forms. Currently, these include pills, pellets and injections, as well as creams, gels, ointments and sublingual lozenges or troches. Before we look at the specific drugs, let's review what is known about the benefits and risks of taking testosterone today.

EFFECT ON BONE

One of the strongest incentives for taking testosterone is the effect it is proving to have on maintaining and restoring bone density in postmenopausal women. Although long-term studies are yet to be completed, shorter studies (two to five years) have been completed. The results are in, reinforcing the medical community's early support of the hormone for treatment of osteoporosis.

As most of us are aware, osteoporosis is a debilitating disease characterized by decreased bone mineral density leading to fractures. Postmenopausal women and elderly men are most commonly affected. Prevention is critical because no drugs are currently available to "mend" or fully restore the damage done to bone by osteoporosis. In fact, one of the first lines of prevention is hormone replacement therapy (HRT).

Several recent and current studies have been devoted to determining just how much of an additional effect testosterone has relative to the positive effect of HRT utilizing estrogen with or without progesterone or a progesteronelike progestogen. As early as 1984 a study cited by Solvay Pharmaceuticals, makers of Estratest, indicated that testosterone can have a powerful effect on bone density. This study found that women with crush fractures of the lower spine had lower levels of androgens (i.e., testosterone) than women without crush fractures.

Over time, the good news has escalated. In December 1999, *The Journal of Reproductive Medicine* reported a two-year study of 311 surgically menopausal women. The women were divided into two groups with one group taking varied doses of estrogen *alone* versus the second group taking varied doses of estrogen *plus testosterone*. A marked difference was found in those who took the estrogen plus testosterone combination.

While all the treatments had prevented *loss* of bone in the spine and hip, the preparations of estrogen plus testosterone *increased spine and hip bone mineral density more than the other treatments—with the highest dosage of testosterone having the greatest effect*. It should be noted, too, that while all the treatments improved menopausal symptoms, those on estrogen plus testosterone also experienced improvement in their sense of well-being and level of sexual interest. Side effects were not significant in either group with no unusual hair growth (hirsutism) reported by any of the women in the study after a full two years.

Underscoring the results of that study was an article by Dr. S. J. Wimalawansa in the summer 2000 issue of the *Journal of Clinical Densitometry* that discussed data from nine other studies on osteoporosis and various HRT therapies. The article stated that three studies showed that "the addition of testosterone to estrogen therapy further increased bone mineral density when compared to estrogen therapy alone, and also prevented the expected decreases in markers of bone formation in early postmenopausal women." The fact bears repeating: Estrogen combined with testosterone *actually increases bone density*.

Another recent study, reported in the September/October 2000 issue of *Menopause*, had similar results. In this study, 57 postmenopausal women who were divided into two groups, one surgical and one natural, took hormone therapy sublingually—one tablet twice a day for one year. (Sublingual means the tablet was absorbed under the tongue, not swallowed. This allows the hormones to bypass the liver and be directly absorbed into the bloodstream.) The women in the study were all in their 54th year and similar in height and weight. Each group was further divided into women taking estrogen alone or taking estrogen with testosterone. Bone density was measured in the anterior-posterior lumbar spine and the total left hip.

After just one year (a short time in the life of a bone!), it was found that while all the groups experienced a *prevention* of bone loss, those taking estrogen with testosterone had *a significant in-*

crease in hip bone mineral density. Curiously, there was no parallel benefit to the spinal bone. This could be attributed to the fact there are two types of bone tissue: cortical bone and trabecular bone. Since the hip is composed of significantly more cortical bone and the spine more of trabecular, this may account for the difference: Testosterone has its most immediate effect on cortical bone tissue. Another factor is that the study was conducted for only one year— a longer period of HRT plus testosterone may have further improved the trabecular bone as well.

Dr. Simon theorizes that testosterone has such a profound effect on bone density for several reasons. Naturally occurring testosterone can be converted to estrogen both in the bloodstream and in bone, leading to higher local levels of estrogen. Testosterone seems to stimulate and maintain bone formation while estrogen stops bone resorption (breakdown). Testosterone can lower sex hormone binding globulin and free up both testosterone (itself) and estrogen. He sees one or more of these effects occurring with both naturally produced testosterone as well as the manufactured methyltestosterone. Having reviewed many more studies than those cited in this chapter, he believes that testosterone acts on bone in even more ways than mentioned here. But if we can slow down bone loss with estrogen and stimulate bone growth with testosterone—we are looking at a powerful tool for preventing osteoporosis.

And this is just the beginning. The positive effect of testosterone on bone ties in to restoring muscle mass as well. Testosterone, like all the androgens, increases lean body mass by helping to convert fat to muscle or, at the very least, by reducing body fat as it increases muscle. This becomes important when you consider that a major health problem among older women is frailty and muscle weakness. By increasing body muscle mass, Simon theorizes, we may be able to improve strength and agility while reducing frailty and a woman's risk profile for fracture.

For example, it's known that frail women have an increased propensity to fall down—and a greater chance of fracturing a bone. On the other hand, women who have better muscle mass or who have more sexually distributed body fat—meaning a little bit of fat around their hips—have more padding in the places they need it. When they fall, they don't break their hips.

So it is that an androgen like testosterone can be used not only to strengthen the bone with bone growth, but it may be also able to strengthen the muscles that would allow for more support around the bone. And reducing the risk of a hip fracture reduces the risk of death because about one-sixth of all patients who experience hip fractures actually die within one year.

It should be noted that androgens other than testosterone such as the androgenic progestins found in Femhrt (norethindrone acetate/ethinyl estradiol) also induce bone formation. Recent studies show that the bone density improvements (about 4–6 percent) induced by the androgenic progestin norethindrone acetate found in Femhrt are similar to the changes seen when methyltestosterone is added to estrogen replacement therapy.

EFFECTS ON THE HEART

While initial tests were encouraging, the effect of androgens, i.e., testosterone, on the cardiovascular health of women remains debatable. Early enthusiasm for the use of testosterone with cardiac patients gave way to negative impressions when it was thought that it might lower "good" cholesterol levels. The jury is still out and numerous studies are under way.

However, one study conducted by physicians in the Netherlands of 45 women with coronary heart disease found that the occurrence of coronary heart disease in middle-aged women was *not* preceded by premenopausal low levels of estrogen and high levels of androgen production. Researchers had launched the study with the belief that testosterone was the culprit and had hypothesized that a high androgen production before menopause might increase the risk for coronary heart disease. This proved not to be the case.

Whatever emerges from new studies and clinical trials over the coming years, it is critical that women, especially older women, remain aware of the newest research on heart disease—whether this involves testosterone or estrogen or any other hormone treatment associated with menopause. A woman is five times more likely to die of a heart attack than she is of breast cancer. And a woman over age 60 is the most at risk.

Why the confusion over the long-term benefit testosterone may have on the heart? Simon explains that it has long been thought that the differences in cardiovascular risk between men and women, with men having greater risk, were related to testosterone. That is much less clear today. For example, we now know that men with *lower*, not *higher* testosterone actually have greater cardiovascular risk. In fact, Simon has seen research indicating that the same conversion of testosterone to estrogen that occurs in bone may also occur within the wall of an artery, particularly a coronary artery. This may mean that the testosterone in men is converted to estrogen in ways that protect them from heart attacks.

However, Simon points out, there is one flaw in that theory.

When testosterone is administered in high doses to men, or when it is given orally to women (in high doses relative to what is appropriate for women), it lowers their HDL, their good cholesterol. This confuses the issue and makes it difficult to reward or blame the androgen for coronary health. Again, Simon underscores that it is exactly this type of contradiction that makes it difficult to assess the long-term benefit to the heart of the postmenopausal woman.

Simon cautions against assuming the worst. A recent study conducted on women *with preexisting heart disease* was interpreted by some in the media to mean that because estrogen did not reverse heart disease, it had no positive effect. Simon argues that that does not answer the important question of primary prevention in women who *do not have a preexisting condition of heart disease*. In other words, we do not yet know if estrogen with or without testosterone—when used early in menopause or just after estrogen levels begin to fall—will reduce the long-term risk of *developing* cardiovascular disease. Though the data isn't in yet, there is enough circumstantial information to encourage that possibility. Testosterone, or its conversion to estradiol, may yet be proven to prevent heart disease in healthy women.

This question of data is a serious one that recurs when looking at all the benefits and risks of testosterone. Relative to the heart, much of the current data is flawed for two reasons: One, it is *only* three years long. And two, the women in some of the studies would not be likely to have had major coronary events just because they're young. For example, if you have a three-year period during which you give a group of 50- to 55-year-old women a drug that increases cholesterol and plaque in their coronary arteries, you wouldn't expect them all to have heart attacks during that three-year period. But if you could follow that group for 15 years, you might see that treating them for three years with the drug had an adverse effect by the time they reached age 65. Obviously, we are years away from having that kind of reliable long-term data.

EFFECTS ON COGNITIVE FUNCTIONING AND MOOD

As more and more information is emerging on the effect of hormones on memory, cognition and mood—both male and female—early results on the benefits of treatment with androgens, specifically testosterone, are encouraging.

We emphasize, however, that these are *early* studies conducted on a limited number of people. It will be years before enough research has been conducted so that conclusions can be definitively drawn.

The following studies are considered preliminary but positive regarding the effect of testosterone on mood and cognitive functioning as well as on libido.

One of the most recent was conducted in 1997 and reported in 1998 by Dr. Simon, along with Drs. Gary G. Kay, Terri Huh, Mark Shepanek, Althea Artis and Brinda Wiita. This team researched the effect of estrogen-testosterone therapy on women who were healthy and surgically menopausal. In the study, twenty-four subjects were given either an estrogen-only (Estratab) ERT or an estrogen-androgen (Estratest) HRT, containing the exact same amount of estrogen. The androgen in Estratest is methyltestosterone.

The women took the HRT for 12 weeks and they were tested twice during this time. The cognitive test battery included measures of math problem solving, spatial rotation, attention span, reaction time and language. In addition, the women were asked to rate their level of sexual desire and mood.

And the results?

On the written math test the Estratest group correctly completed 1.3 more problems per two minutes than the Estratab group; and on the spatial rotation test, these subjects demonstrated *twice as much improvement* in the number of problems solved per minute as compared to the subjects taking estrogen alone.

Those receiving Estratest expressed *significantly less* inhibition of sexual desire. This was in sharp contrast to those taking the estrogen-only Estratab who demonstrated no effect on sexual desire. The enhanced sexual functioning and mood led to significantly stronger feelings of "improvement in quality of life" for the Estratest group as well.

And the conclusion? "The addition of androgen to estrogen appears to be beneficial to sexual desire and to specific cognitive functions," stated the final paper.

A number of studies were reviewed in an article published by the University of Western Australia Department of Psychiatry and Behavioural Science, which noted that data on the effect of testosterone on postmenopausal women is "sparse" but preliminary findings "suggest that testosterone therapy may improve mood when used in isolation or in association with estrogen . . . some studies indicate that the administration of testosterone . . . is associated with better visuospatial functioning and . . . verbal skills."

Yet another study, reported in *Neurology*, February 2000, by researchers from the Graduate School of Psychology at Fuller Theological Seminary in Pasedena, California, found that "levels of testosterone were related positively to verbal fluency." The authors of this study measured "circulating sex hormone levels in 39 highly educated, nondemented, predominantly white elderly women."

And a study that was reported in the March 1999 issue of the *American Journal of Obstetrics & Gynecology* by Dr. P. M. Sarrel of Yale University also held some good news. This article said, "Results from clinical studies show that hormone replacement therapy with estrogen plus androgens provides greater improvement in psychologic (e.g., lack of concentration, depression and fatigue) and sexual (e.g., decreased libido and inability to have an orgasm) symptoms than does estrogen alone in naturally and surgically menopausal women."

It should be noted that among the androgenic drugs that look promising is Femhrt (norethindrone acetate/ethinyl estradiol), which features androgenic progestogen norethindrone acetate added to the ethinyl estradiol. Femhrt has been shown in preliminary studies to improve libido and sense of well-being much like the true androgens (i.e., testosterone). More studies are underway.

Dr. Simon adds to that the fact that men get far less Alzheimer's disease than women. And women get far less heart disease than men. The hypothesis is that men get less Alzheimer's because their levels of testosterone persist in their blood until they're very old, certainly into their 90s. Since we know that testosterone can be converted to estrogen, we assume that estrogen is good for prevention of Alzheimer's. Again, as with heart disease, we mean "primary prevention." That is, people without Alzheimer's disease who are given estrogen appear to have less risk of getting Alzheimer's disease.

However, the most recent data, just like that for heart disease, suggests that individuals *with* Alzheimer's disease who receive estrogen do not significantly improve. And it may be that estrogen, or testosterone converted into estrogen, is an edge that men have over women because their testosterone level doesn't drop at age 50 to 55 as it does in women—a few years following menopause. Instead, the big pool of testosterone that they have well into their 90s is easily converted to estrogen in the brain, preventing Alzheimer's and explaining the large difference in its incidence in women and men.

Mood enhancement also raises questions. While testosterone has been shown to enhance mood, particularly as it relates to energy and well-being, it has also been shown to increase sexual fantasies and arousal. However, points out Simon, all of those studies suffer from the same two problems.

One problem is that they were all done in surgically menopausal women. While that's a good model for studying testosterone's effect, because all the testosterone is coming from the treatment rather than from the woman, the studies can and have been criticized. It is difficult to prove that the testosterone did more than bring the level of enhancement—whether that is energy level or sense of well-being—from a below-normal level to a normal level. So it may not be an enhancement but a restoration to normal. That's one possibility. The other criticism is that the studies used a very high dose of testosterone, one that today would be considered supraphysiologic. And the question is: Were these effects physiologic or pharmacologic, a function of the body or a function of the drug? And that is not yet resolved.

Separate from Dr. Simon's findings, I would like to add that every one of the women taking testosterone and interviewed for this book, including myself, said we felt a marked enhancement in our mood and energy levels once we started taking the hormone. It should be taken into consideration that some of the women take antidepressants. But I do not take an antidepressant, nor do a number of the women who said they experienced these positive, healthy feelings. While ours may be subjective responses not documented by years of medical research, they are still important because we feel better than we did *before taking testosterone.*

EFFECTS ON BODY FAT, MUSCLE STRENGTH AND MUSCLE MASS

Menopause has been associated with the loss of skeletal mass, lean body mass and an increase in fat, particularly abdominal fat. The more time that passes after menopause, the greater the increase in weight as well as in the total and the percentage of body fat. The loss of lean body mass is believed to increase the risk of developing diseases such as osteoporosis, while the increase in abdominal fat has been linked to increased cardiovascular risk, insulin resistance and diabetes.

This was the background for a recent study comparing the effect of taking estrogen alone versus taking a combination of estrogen with testosterone. The study was conducted by Adrian S. Dobs, M.D., M.H.S.; Tam Nguyen, B.S.; and Cindy Pace, B.S.; and the results were reported in March 2001 as "The Differential Effects of Oral Estrogen versus Oral-Estrogen-Androgen Replacement Therapy on Body Composition in Postmenopausal Women."

These researchers studied 40 women who were either surgically or naturally menopausal with a mean age of 57 years and a mean weight of 157 pounds. The mean time since menopause was ten years and all the women had received hormone replacement therapy longer than one year. In order to participate in the study, the women were required to have been on estrogen replacement therapy for at least three months and to have normal liver and renal function tests and serum lipids. Half the group took estrogen alone and half took a combination of estrogen with testosterone.

The results showed that four months of estrogen-testosterone therapy *increased* lean body mass and muscle strength. It also showed statistically significant reductions in the percentage of body fat. Secondary objectives of the study were to assess changes in sexual function, quality of life and cardiovascular risk factors. Based on questionnaires they completed during different stages of the study, the estrogen-testosterone group showed significant improvement in sexual functioning, including increased interest in sex and other beneficial changes in factors used to measure quality of life. Since excess body fat is a strong cardiovascular risk factor, the participants' increase in lean body mass is a positive result. No notable side effects were reported.

It should be understood, however, that any long-term effects on the liver are not clear from this short-term study.

Testosterone: The Side Effects

I assume the risk of potential side effects from using this hormone. All the women I've interviewed and who are taking testosterone are also well aware that they are taking risks.

What are these risks? The only complaint that I have had and that I have heard most frequently is this: a modest increase in hair growth. This means shaving our legs more frequently, plucking random dark hairs from our chins or upper lips, and, for a few, bleaching the fine hair growth on the upper lip.

However, note that we are all taking testosterone under the care of a physician. Our hormone replacement therapy is prescribed for each of us individually. No one takes more than she needs, which is why the only negative side effect we experience is the modest hair growth.

Simon sees patients who have not been so careful. A look at what is to be expected versus extreme reactions will help you gauge what is likely to occur with your use of testosterone in hormone replacement therapy.

A reassuring note here is that the side effects resulting from increased testosterone levels or androgen replacement therapy are very easily recognized—they do not sneak up on you. For example, when you are a teenager, it is the change in your androgens (i.e., an increase in testosterone) that causes oily skin, acne and hair growth. This includes pubic hair. Identical side effects will occur with testosterone replacement therapy—and the degree to which they appear will depend on the dosage and the duration of use.

Individuals who use a very high dose of testosterone for a short period of time may have no side effects whatsoever. Those who use a high dose for a long period of time will have more side effects than if they used a high dose for an intermediate period of time. *It is the individual who uses a low dose for a long period of time that experiences the least amount of side effects—ranging from none at all to mild.*

Any side effects that are going to occur are most likely to be seen with the initiation of androgen replacement therapy. The first of these is acne because the sebaceous glands, those glands in the skin that make oil and erupted when you were a teenager, are typically not very active in a postmenopausal woman. Since they have not been stimulated for a while, they have a tendency to have become plugged with normal skin cell debris. When a woman starts taking an androgen after ten or 15 years of relative inactivity, the glands tend to wake up and cause some acne. But once the pores get cleaned out, the normal lanolin of the body is restored and the acne disappears. Now the woman feels like her skin is softer, more supple, even thicker—which may be the result of both estrogen and testosterone.

An interesting aside to this change in skin tone is the effect it has psychologically. Because a postmenopausal woman typically suffers from dry skin, she is a high consumer of moisturizers and other lanolin-based skin products. Consequently, she associates this change in her skin with being more youthful, more like it was when she was in her 30s and early 40s. Once taking testosterone, she often ends up using less moisturizer or none at all!

Initially, then, a woman may have acne but it is likely to be very short-term, especially because the dosage of testosterone is in a "normal" physiologic range. *Remember, cautions Simon, all we're doing is restoring levels to what they were when the women were younger. We're not trying to give them more than they had.*

However, if there is long-term exposure to *excessive* levels, there will be a related increase in hair. The hair could be a normal pattern of hair distribution for an adult woman—new growth on her underarms, her legs, and her pubic area. But if there is too much testosterone, then the hair growth may resemble normal distribution for a man—hair on the chin or the upper lip or some combination.

Keep in mind that there are major differences between different ethnic groups in what passes for "normal" facial and body hair. For example, Mediterranean women have much more dark hair on the face and upper lip and sideburn areas than is found in women from Scandinavia or Asia. The latter tend to have very little body hair. It is important to remember these differences before ascribing any changes in the amount of new hair growth as being a negative rather than a restorative result.

Most of the time, if the dosage of testosterone is appropriate and the levels in the blood are within a normal physiologic range, there is very little effect on body hair that cannot be explained as being normal or restorative to premenopausal amounts.

Given that it is very common for women to have some mild acne, some increase in the oiliness of skin and some change in new hair growth during the first three months of androgen replacement therapy, it is crucial to pay close attention to these changes as they determine the correct levels of testosterone a woman needs. The reason for this is that adding testosterone to hormone replacement therapy—in the forms currently available—presents a challenge in "fine-tuning" for the individual.

Simon underscores the need to monitor even modest changes. No matter how expert the physician is at determining the correct testosterone replacement, the drugs available to date have not been as good as they need to be.

Many times during the course of a month or three months when he is starting a patient out on hormone replacement therapy, she may be getting more than she needs. And that is one of the major advantages of a new testosterone patch, which is still in clinical trials. The patch can be cut and tailored to provide the exact dose wanted and the compound itself (natural testosterone) can be measured very accurately in blood because it's delivered at a steady rate instead of bouncing up and down. This allows a physician to measure it in the blood after a woman has been on the patch for a defined period of time—usually four to six weeks—and know exactly how much testosterone she has in her bloodstream. It also makes it possible for the physician to adjust the dosage and keep it in a range that is normal for that particular woman. It all adds up to minimizing side effects—including those random hairs. (We'll say more about this new patch in the next section of this chapter where we discuss current and new drugs.)

While the most common side effects are minor when a woman is careful with the amount of androgen she is taking and she is doing so under the care of a physician, the woman who is not careful can run into serious problems. Simon has seen many instances when testosterone was given in significantly elevated amounts, not monitored carefully, or when women self-administered.

The woman who takes it upon herself to take more testosterone than prescribed by a physician is making a serious mistake. She may do so because she feels better, has more energy, is more sexual, her orgasms are more intense, etc., etc., but what she has done is use way too much. In cases like that, Simon has seen women lose much of the hair on their heads, particularly temporal balding or balding in general. They may experience voice changes due to a thickening of the vocal cords and loss of voice in the high registers. Those two changes—hair loss and a deepening of the voice—are rare but when he sees these signs, Simon has found they are almost always related to excessive dosing. Fortunately, most of these side effects are reversible.

A final side effect is a decrease in the level of body fat. It has long been known that testosterone lowers the amount of body fat as it increases lean body mass. If the testosterone dose is in the normal range, there will be no major change in body fat *distribution*, only in the *amount*. But if you use excessive doses of testosterone, a woman can get very muscular. You see this in elite athletes or professional bodybuilders who have little or no body fat, but that is an extraordinary loss that occurs only with high doses of the androgen.

Recognize that muscle weighs more than fat. Some patients become alarmed, especially at first, when they find their weight is going up—but become exceedingly pleased when, despite the increase in weight, their dress size may be smaller.

Most of Simon's patients receiving a normal range of testosterone are pleased with a reasonable and beneficial effect on their body fat. Both physician and patient stay alert for changes, however, as any more than a "reasonable" change may signal that the individual is taking too much testosterone.

Testosterone Options

A physician has a variety of options for prescribing testosterone. As we stated earlier, however, the existing FDA-approved drugs "are not as good as they need to be." That's why, after describing each, we'll look at the drawbacks of that particular form or compound.

PILLS

In pill form designed to be taken orally are Estratest and Estratest H.S. (half-strength). Manufactured by Solvay, these pills are available in two methyltestosterone dosages, 1.25 mg. and 2.5 mg. Generically, the drug is identified as "esterified estrogens and methyltestosterone." Estratest H.S. has the same generic name and is manufactured by Solvay in dosages of 0.625mg. and 1.25 mg.

The chief drawbacks of the pills are that they limit the amount of testosterone that can be taken and they are metabolized through the liver. Many women need a hormone therapy that will bypass the liver because oral testosterone may reduce or negate the effect estrogens have on their body chemistry. The reasons for this are complex and underscore why it is essential never to self-administer any androgen.

On the other hand, a recent study on Estratest was very reassuring. After two years of use, a very small percentage of women on the lower dose Estratest H.S. found that their hair growth, acne or skin was no more affected by taking an estrogen-testosterone drug than it was when they took only estrogen. There was, it should be noted, a modest increase in the number of women reporting symptoms among those who took the higher dose Estratest. Similarly, Femhrt's androgenic progestins seldom cause negative effects.

INJECTIONS

Depo-Testadiol is administered by injection. The generic name of this drug is "testosterone cypionate/estradiol cypionate." Manufactured by Pharmacia & Upjohn, it is available in dosages of testosterone 50 mg. estradiol 2 mg./ml.

Delatestryl is an injection whose generic name is "testosterone enanthate." It is manufactured by BTG and available in dosages of 200mg./ml.

Depo-Testosterone is an injection whose generic name is "testosterone cypionate." It is manufactured by Star in dosages of 200mg./ml.

"The injectable testosterones—which are testosterone enanthate, testosterone propionate, and testosterone cypionate—are available as generics from a variety of manufacturers."

One advantage of injections is that a physician can regulate and monitor when they are given and how much is given. Also, the injection goes pretty much directly into the bloodstream, bypassing the liver. The difficulties are twofold: First, it requires an appointment with the doctor and the attendant expense. Second, in order to get a relatively stable amount in the blood for a reasonable period of time, such as a month, you have to give too much at the beginning in order to get enough at the end. So you have to overdose a woman with a testosterone injection in order to get enough in the blood to remain there for a reasonable period of time between injections—ultimately risking unwanted side effects.

PELLETS

Testopel is a pellet whose generic name is "testosterone." It is manufactured by Bartor in a dose of 75 mg.

Other testosterone implants or pellets are manufactured by a variety of formulating pharmacies including the College Pharmacy in a dose of 75 mg.

Subcutaneous testosterone pellets have been used for about 50 years. They're usually given with estradiol pellets because if you're going to have one pellet inserted you might as well have both. They are commonly used in England, Europe, Australia and New Zealand.

The major advantages are twofold: First, they bypass the liver;

and, second, they provide nice stable levels for four to six months. The disadvantages are also twofold: not only do you risk "overdosing" during the early months, but a minor surgical procedure is required to insert them. The surgery means that you must see your doctor two to three times a year, which makes this option more expensive.

CREAMS, GELS AND OINTMENTS

Generically named, "formulated testosterone in petroleum" is a cream that is pharmacy formulated in doses of one percent to two percent.

Also generically named is "formulated testosterone in APC," a cream that is pharmacy formulated in doses of four percent to eight percent. These are the non-oral compounds most frequently used by Simon in his practice.

It is not news that testosterone can be administered as a cream, gel or ointment that is applied locally on the genitals, clitoris or anywhere on the skin. The problem is that they have a tremendous potential for abuse. Physicians find that it is not uncommon for an individual to believe that if a little is good, a little more is better.

Simon has seen innumerable cases of women who self-administered testosterone in this form and who, over the course of time, increased their dose to the point where they ended up with very high levels in their blood. They consequently had extreme and significant side effects. Full beards. Balding. Changes in their voice. Loss of subcutaneous fat around the breasts and hips so that they looked like a man.

In addition to the side effects—if they have used excessive

amounts, their bodies become accustomed to much higher levels so that even lowering their dose results in deficiencies. For example, a woman whose libido and sexual functioning is satisfied with very high doses of testosterone may become sexually dysfunctional on supraphysiologic levels of testosterone once her body has become accustomed to the very high doses. Her thermostat has been reset at an artificially high level.

SUBLINGUAL

The final parenteral (meaning "nonoral") option is a tablet or lozenge held under the tongue that is absorbed directly into the bloodstream. Current versions are compounded by a pharmacy. Simon does not prescribe any sublingual versions of generic testosterone but is aware that several sublingual drugs are in development. While the advantage is the ability for the androgen to bypass the liver, the current sublingual drugs have several disadvantages not the least of which is they taste bad. They are absorbed very quickly and disappear quickly, which leads to a woman having to take more than she needs in order to have any effect. Also, they are not FDA-approved.

MIXING AND MATCHING

Often no single option is satisfactory. Simon has found that most women who walk into his office have already seen one or several gynecologists and have already tried all the available options. This is where "fine-tuning" enters the picture.

He explains the process: "By the time they get to me they've tried Estratest, maybe five or six different estrogens, and many have even tried some over-the-counter preparations. We begin by revisiting everything they've tried because often they may not have used it long enough or in a dose that's adequate to what they need."

For example, a woman who has been on hormone replacement therapy for less than a month at a particular dose probably has not reached a steady state on that preparation and cannot possibly know if it's going to work or not. But if that criteria is met and libido continues to be the main issue, then Simon is likely to prescribe three monthly injections.

"I do this knowing that I'm going to overdose them on testosterone because most of the time, I do not believe that their problem is *solely* hormonal," said Simon. "These are patients who have already seen other physicians and have tried several other medications.

"By giving a very well understood, although partially excessive, dose of testosterone for a period of three months, one thing becomes clear," he explains. "If they do not have a reasonable response to their symptoms, then testosterone is not going to work. This is how I separate those patients with exclusively hormonally dependent problems from those who have psychological, social or relationship issues. And it works. At the end of three months, the women who have a solely hormonal problem tell me they are great. In fact, they tell me their husbands or partners can't keep up with them and they could use—'just a little less.' "

At this point, Simon will cut the dose or switch them to a different option. "I don't like to keep a woman on long-term injections because it can have too many side effects and be too expensive. I prefer a form of testosterone replacement therapy that can be used long-term. Usually, the choice is Estratest, which may not have worked in the past but it does now. Why? Because the woman now knows that her body *can* work, it just needs a boost."

While Simon feels Estratest is the best option for low dosages over the long term, there is an alternative. In selective cases, he will prescribe testosterone in a cream that can be applied to the pubic area and the clitoris. Or he will tell them to use Estratest until the new testosterone patch or other options in development become available.

As demonstrated, this "mixing and matching" is a process that takes place over a period ranging from three months to a year. The challenge for the physician and the patient is to find the particular hormone balance that is calibrated to her body chemistry and her health care needs.

New Testosterone Drugs in Development

We have referred several times now to "the new testosterone patch." Before we take a close look at that, here is a brief review of a myriad of new testosterone and androgen products in the "research and development" pipeline. Following this list, we will examine the patch more closely because it is in the final stage of clinical trials and is due to be approved for use soon.

The drugs that follow are still in the early stages of development. Since most pharmaceuticals prefer to avoid detailed descriptions before new drugs reach the market, including naming their product, our information is limited. However, it helps to know how much emphasis there is on finding new testosterone and androgen drugs—these billions of research dollars would not be spent if medical and health experts did not believe that millions of men and women need these products.

Research and clinical studies are under way on two categories of treatment: hormone therapy designed to restore desire; and other drugs designed to increase or amplify the sensations of arousal.

Among the companies currently developing drugs to restore desire are these: Organon is in trials with "Livial" (tibolone); Noven is developing an androgen/estrogen combination patch; Unimed is developing two androgen products, a di hydro testosterone gel called Andractin and a testosterone gel called ReLibra; Cellegy is working on a testosterone gel called Tostrelle; and Galen Holdings is developing a testosterone-containing vaginal ring. Watson is working on an FDA-approved formulation of DHEA and Novavax is developing a testosterone lotion to be called Androsorb and an estradiol/testosterone combination lotion called Test-ESTRA-SORB.

In the rush to develop drugs designed to increase blood flow and heighten sensation (similar to Viagra) for both men and women, the following are in development for possible use by women: Pfizer is working on a Viagra for women (sildenafil citrate); Bayer is working on a similar compound called Vardenifil; Zonagen is developing phentolamine (Vasomax); Eli Lilly has a joint venture with Icos on a compound known as Cialis; NexMed is working on Femprox, a cream formulation of alprostadil; and Harvard Scientific on a similar prostoglandin. Vivus is also working on a prostoglandin cream called Alista and TAP on apomorphine (Uprima). Finally, Sepracor is developing an isomer of the diet drug Sibutramine (Meridia), which appears to have sexual arousal–inducing properties.

As stated earlier, these are in development and may be years away from reaching the market. And by the time you read this, half a dozen more may be in development.

THE BEST OF THE NEW: THE TRANSDERMAL PATCH

The first question to ask is why a *patch*? Why something that adheres to the outside of your body in order to do its job inside?

Because medicating through the skin rather than by needle, pellet or through the stomach has many advantages.

For example, not only do needles hurt but—when it comes to administering testosterone— both injections and pellets require expensive interaction in the doctor's office.

Pills have disadvantages, too. Not only are they limited in the amount of testosterone they can deliver, but when drugs are swallowed, their molecules tend to charge out of the stomach or the intestine into the bloodstream—fast acting, instantly at work. Their absorption may be highly variable and further affected by food or drink. Alternatively, they are rushed to the liver where their molecular structure may be changed by the liver's enzymes, then they charge out into the rest of the body. While this is great for antibiotics where fast action is necessary to work best, drugs like hormones do their work much better on a slower schedule, a schedule that lets them take effect without structural changes and at low levels over a long period of time.

It is exactly this pattern that is ideal for testosterone. Avoiding the structural change that can take place in the liver works well for those women sensitive to estrogens. In addition, the patch allows the careful calibration of low levels of hormone over a long period of time. This helps a physician avoid the "overdosing" of testosterone that is inherent in the use of an injection or a pellet.

Best of all, a woman does not have to see a doctor every few months for another pellet or monthly injection. Our skin acts like a high-quality raincoat letting small molecules of powerful drugs seep through to work in very low concentrations over time.

This ability to carefully control the androgen explains the enthusiastic response the medical community has had to news that a "transdermal" testosterone skin patch has been shown to markedly improve sexual functioning and a sense of well-being in surgically menopausal women. The patch is in the final pivotal clinical trials and may be FDA-approved and available soon.

Simon was a member of the six-person team of research physicians conducting the clinical trials that resulted in this breakthrough. Even though the studies were done on surgically menopausal women, the ramifications can eventually be applied to women who are naturally menopausal and whose hormones show greater fluctuation.

A synopsis of the study was issued by Massachusetts General Hospital, the large teaching hospital affiliated with Harvard Medical School, while a paper detailing the study was published in the September 7, 2000, issue of the *New England Journal of Medicine*. We would like to share highlights of the synopsis of the study as this transdermal patch is likely to be a significant new option for postmenopausal women.

First, the project was conducted nationally and involved a

multi-institutional research group led by researchers from Massachusetts General Hospital (MGH), Proctor & Gamble Company and Watson Laboratories, Inc., a division of Watson Pharmaceuticals. Their conclusion stated that they "found that use of an experimental testosterone skin patch can relieve impaired sexual functioning in . . . women who have had their ovaries removed before natural menopause."

"We know that women who have gone through menopause after surgical removal of their ovaries have decreased testosterone levels," said Jan Shifren, M.D., of MGH and the paper's lead author. "This study indicates that women who have experienced a loss of sexual functioning after such surgery may benefit from returning their testosterone levels to normal through use of a testosterone skin patch."

The synopsis explains, as we have earlier in this book, that women normally produce testosterone in their ovaries and adrenal glands and may require sufficient levels of the hormone for proper sexual functioning. About half a woman's testosterone comes from the ovaries—so those whose ovaries are removed before menopause lose about half their natural testosterone, along with 80 percent of their natural estrogens. While estrogen replacement therapy can relieve symptoms such as hot flashes, vaginal atrophy and osteoporosis in these women, many who take estrogen still report a loss of sexual desire, activity and pleasure as well as a reduced overall sense of well-being.

Given that detail, it was pointed out by Norm Mazer, M.D., Ph.D., senior medical research fellow at Watson Laboratories and the study's designer, that the project differed from other efforts in a critical way: "This study was built on the work of earlier researchers who first recognized the potential of testosterone to improve sexual functioning in women after surgical menopause. But these earlier studies treated women with testosterone injections or implants, which resulted in higher than normal serum testosterone levels. The testosterone patches developed by Watson Laboratories were specifically designed to restore testosterone levels to the normal range of healthy young women."

The study involved 75 women, ages 31 to 56, each of whom had undergone a hysterectomy and an oophorectomy anywhere from one to ten years before the study began. All had testosterone levels that were below average in comparison to healthy young women, and despite daily oral estrogen replacement therapy, all reported having less active or less satisfying sex lives as compared with before their surgery. In fact, each had been in a stable, monogamous heterosexual relationship for at least one year.

During the 36-week study, the women went through three consecutive 12-week treatment periods during which they received, in random order, three combinations of skin patches. The patches delivered daily doses of either 300 micrograms of testosterone, 150 micrograms of testosterone, or a placebo. Neither the participants nor the investigators working with them knew which patch combinations the women were receiving at any time.

Each woman completed an evaluation of sexual functioning—including desire, arousal, activity and pleasure—as well as an evaluation of overall psychological well-being at the beginning of the study and at the end of each treatment period. Her testosterone levels were measured at four-week intervals, and each participant continued to receive oral estrogen replacement therapy during this time.

In the end, authoritative data was gathered from 65 study participants (ten dropped out for a variety of reasons not related to the treatment). The women reported increased sexual activity and pleasure in all three treatment periods, including placebo, *but significantly greater improvement was seen at the 300 microgram dose level compared to placebo.*

The women also reported improved overall psychological well-being with treatment. Adverse side effects of the type often associated with excess testosterone levels were not reported at significant levels. Most important, the levels of HDL cholesterol, the so-called "good cholesterol," were not lowered by transdermal testosterone treatment.

Testosterone levels remained low during placebo periods but rose to midnormal and high-normal levels when women received the 150- and 300-microgram doses, respectively. The testosterone treatment had no effect on their estrogen levels.

The researchers noted that even women receiving placebo doses reported improved sexual functioning compared with their experiences before starting the study. Several factors could explain this response. These include the women's strong motivation to improve their sex lives, their improved communication with their sexual partners, the presence of the patches as a visible reminder of the treatment's goal, and the continuation of patterns of greater sexual activity that began when the women were receiving active doses.

However surprising the response was to the placebo, the numbers told the story: The higher testosterone dose of 300 micrograms improved sexual functioning and psychological well-being substantially more than the lower dose or the placebo effect.

Speaking of numbers, it is important to note the scope of the researchers and authors of the study. Their expertise and the support of their institutions underscore the value this study has for women.

Participants in the research and coauthors of the article in the *New England Journal of Medicine*—in addition to Shifren, Mazer and Simon—were Glenn Braunstein, M.D., of Cedars-Sinai Medical Center in Los Angeles; Peter Casson, M.D., and John Buster, M.D., of Baylor College of Medicine, Houston; Geoffrey Redmond, M.D., and Regina Burki, M.D., of Salt Lake City; Elizabeth Ginsburg, M.D., of Brigham and Women's Hospital, Boston; Raymond Rosen, Ph.D., and Sandra Leiblum, Ph.D., of Robert Woods Johnson Medical School in New Jersey; Kim Caramelli, M.S., of Watson Pharmaceuticals, Utah; Kirtley Jones, M.D., of University of Utah Medical Center in Salt Lake City; and Clair Daugherty, M.S., of Anesta Corporation in Salt Lake City.

Why do we feel such a study is so important? Not only do 600,000 women have hysterectomies annually—with nearly as many losing their ovaries as well—but recent medical survey data suggests that *nearly 40 percent of American women experience sexual dysfunction.*

Dr. Simon and I feel there is no longer any good reason why so many women should have to feel as if they have lost an essential part of themselves. It is time that women understand how they can restore their passion for life, restore themselves.

In the next chapter we will help you decide if you are one of these women and, if you are, how to talk to your physician and change your life.

Eight

The Testosterone Decision:
How to Find, Talk and Work with
Your Doctor

If some of the personal stories in the earlier chapters alarm you, making it seem as if menopause takes over and dismantles your life, that's not true. What is disturbing is the lack of information and understanding of what is changing as you experience menopause. Keep in mind that almost all of the women profiled had difficulty finding physicians who could help them, not to mention finding current and easy-to-read information about androgens like testosterone. If you've read the chapters in this book that relate to your situation, you already know more than those women did just a few years ago. You know more than many doctors.

This chapter is designed to give you a quick review of important points that will help you find, talk and work with your doctor. Dr. Simon and I will also recommend resources you can use to find the latest information on testosterone.

The Most Frequently Asked Questions

Q: If my regular ob-gyn is resistant to combination estrogen-testosterone therapy, how can I find a doctor who will help me? And why are so many doctors resistant to this therapy?

A: Let's tackle the "resistance" issue first. It's one that I have dealt with personally.

You'll recall from the Introduction that my longtime ob-gyn, a woman, initially told me my problem was "in your head." She did an abrupt about-face when I presented her with contrary information a year later. She's not the only doctor with whom I had difficulty. Three years later, I moved to a university town in Missouri and made an appointment with an ob-gyn, a man, who was highly recommended by several women. I explained the estrogen-replacement therapy that I had been taking and my wish to continue with Estratest and Provera. He gave me a new prescription, but said as he handed it to me, *"Now don't you tell anyone else I'm giving you this."* He made it clear he thought I was doing something wrong.

In sharp contrast is the positive attitude of my current ob-gyn, a man in his late 30s, who I see here in northern Wisconsin. The fact that this is a rural region does not mean our medical community is less informed. Instead, my ob-gyn has a broad patient base of women who are both pre- and postmenopausal. During our first visit, he listened to what I had to say about my hormone therapy and renewed my prescription with enthusiasm. A highlight of my annual checkup is our discussion of the newest information on the subject. Should I experience any side effects or symptoms that concern me, I have confidence that my physician is either informed or willing to seek out the information needed. This is what you want.

THE RESISTANT PHYSICIAN

But why are so many doctors resistant to estrogen-testosterone therapy? Why do so many prescribe *just one hormone therapy for all their patients*? Why do they seem so unwilling to work with you to find exactly the right combination for your body chemistry?

Solvay Pharmaceuticals, makers of Estratest, recently conducted interviews with 21 physicians, to explore these questions. Here is what they learned.

The single most important reason for physician resistance is *lack of education*. Very few understood the role that androgens, such as testosterone, play in female physiology or the direct effects these hormones have on the various organ systems already discussed. They were not aware that the normal reproductive-age woman has higher circulating levels of androgens (testosterone in particular) than estrogen virtually every day of her menstrual cycle. Consequently, they said they had no reason to prescribe androgens for women whether premenopausal or postmenopausal.

Their experience and training is to replace estrogen only and to give the postmenopausal women WITH A UTERUS a progestogen, like progesterone only to protect the uterus from the estrogen. And even then—in a busy managed-care one-size-fits-all world, they said it takes "too much time" to work on other issues besides controlling general menopausal symptoms and preventing osteoporosis. If one formulation of estrogen or one product can solve those basic problems in most of their patients that's enough for them. It may also be important that many physicians and other health care providers feel uncomfortable talking about sex and interpersonal relationship issues. They know if you bring up the subject of androgens that SEX is the next subject. In a small town, where everyone knows everyone, this may be a particular problem.

Again, because of their lack of education, they are uninformed of the actual effects of low doses of androgens. Basing their opinions on obsolete data reviewed years ago, they are afraid of causing virilising side effects (i.e., unwanted hair and voice changes) even though *they have not seen any such side effects* in the rare instances when they have prescribed an estrogen-androgen product such as Estratest or Femhrt. They are unwilling or unable to balance that concern with the potential benefits. Because of their lack of education, they may be unaware of the benefits and just how safe the appropriate doses of testosterone can be.

It should be noted that these physicians are not always encouraged to update their medical education by their national associations either. The American College of Obstetricians & Gynecologists (ACOG) failed to recognize the importance of several new studies on the use of androgens in female hormone replacement therapy and recently recommended against replacing testosterone in women.

Another opinion on physician resistance was mentioned by one of Proctor & Gamble's research experts who said, "A big problem is that 30-year-old intern who can't imagine his mother wanting to have sex . . ."

We can view these attitudes as laziness or as ignorance, but we have to look at the reality: The burden of our health care rests on the shoulders of one party—**ourselves.**

Q: I understand what you say about a physician's reluctance to prescribe androgens but I'm unsure what to do. I've been seeing the same ob-gyn for many years. My doctor knows me and knows my body. Except for this issue, I trust my doctor's opinion. Must I change physicians?

A: If you have a long-term patient-doctor relationship that you are hesitant to terminate, we suggest you ask your ob-gyn if they would refer you to a colleague who is specializing in hormone replacement therapies or has a particular interest in the consequences of menopause. Such physicians may have a variety of different backgrounds. While most are likely to be obstetricians and gynecologists, others may be trained as internists or family physicians, they may be subspecialized in medical endocrinology or like Dr. Simon, reproductive endocrinology. Some may not be physicians at all. Many interested and well-trained individuals can be midwives, physician assistants and nurse practitioners. Make sure your physician realizes he or she is referring you *for a consultation* or *second opinion* only; this will reassure him or her that you are not bailing out of a long-term therapeutic relationship—only that you are interested in more information. Suggest that your doctor coordinate your care with your hormone therapy. Make it clear that this is of great importance to you, that you are aware this is a new area of medicine and you are not critical of your current care. This gives you the opportunity to explore your options for hormone therapy while maintaining contact with your regular ob-gyn.

Q: I need to find a physician who can help me decide whether estrogen-testosterone therapy is right for me. Where can I find referrals?

A: The North American Menopause Society (NAMS) is a fine resource. The Society offers the latest information on menopause treatment as well as lists of physicians in your area specializing in menopause.

Web site: www.menopause.org

E-mail: info@menopause.org

Automated Consumer Request Line: 800-774-5342

Phone: 440-442-7550 and Fax: 440-442-2660

Another suggestion is to tackle the Web for sites where professional papers and the latest studies are available to the medical community. Often you can contact the doctors listed on articles found in respected medical journals. Most articles now include e-mail addresses and researchers can be surprisingly responsive. They may be able to recommend individual physicians or a professional society in your region for a referral. If they don't have e-mail, call directory assistance and contact the doctor directly.

Your public library may be able to help you locate these sites and here are several you can try:

To reach the National Library of Medicine, call 1-888-FINDNLM or go to www.nlm.nih.gov. Once there, you can search by subject matter.

To reach the medical journal database Medline, go to www. medlineplus.gov or you can go to the Houston Academy of Medicine–Texas Medical Center Library (www.library.tmc.edu) where librarians will help you.

And, finally, a popular service—but one that charges a fee for referrals—is Best Doctors, which has a database of doctors rated by their peers as the top experts in their field. For more information see www.bestdoctors.com or call 1-888-DOCTORS.

Q: I am about to visit my doctor to discuss hormone therapy. How should I prepare?

A: You will need a complete medical history, including all major health events in your life and a list of any current medications you may be using. A health history of family members with any type of cancer, cardiovascular problems and any other significant health problems is needed as well.

Make a list of your physical symptoms. The following should help you.

GENERAL HEALTH

Contrast your current state of health with how you were five or ten years ago. Begin by assessing your sense of well-being.

- Is your energy level low?

- Do you feel a lack of vitality?

- Do you feel more anxious than is normal for you?

- Have you experienced recent weight gain?

- A loss of muscle tone and muscle strength?

- Dry skin and/or dry scalp?

- Loss of hair, thinning pubic hair or any unusual hair growth?

- Concern over memory and/or lack of mental sharpness?

- If you are not menopausal, do you have a history of your mother's health and experience with menopause? Specifically, at what age did she enter menopause and what were her symptoms? This can be helpful as some of our health patterns are genetic in origin.

SEXUAL HEALTH

The following questions will help you and your doctor determine if you may be experiencing some sexual dysfunction as a result of a testosterone deficiency in addition to the usual symptoms of menopause. As you review each question, ask yourself, *Does it make me unhappy? Is this causing me personal distress? If that is the case, emphasize that in your discussion with the doctor.*

- Are you currently taking any antidepressants? Among those that are likely to cause depressed libido or other sexual problems are the SSRIs, medications like Prozac, Zoloft and Paxil. Recent studies, reported in *The Wall Street Journal*, have shown that between 30 percent and 60 percent of patients taking these drugs experience some form of sexual dysfunction, ranging from loss of desire to problems with arousal and an inability to reach orgasm. This is true for both men and women. Also, keep in the back of your mind that you are likely taking one of these medications for depression, obsessive/compulsive disorder or another such problem, and many of these disorders have sexual problems as part of the syndrome.

- Ask yourself which came first, the chicken or the egg: Did the sexual problem start before the treatment or after? This approach can often help understand the cause, but often it can be very difficult to separate the different causes.

- Do you feel different, sexually, than you did when you were younger? If you have experienced a loss of desire or libido, can you remember when that started?

- Are you having fewer sexual thoughts, dreams or fantasies than you did as a young woman?

- If you masturbated then, do you still? As frequently—or not at all?

- In the past, did you usually respond to sexual cues or advances from men or women who attracted you? Do you still? Do you respond in the same way?

- Do you feel sexual desire for your partner? As often as you want to? When did this change?

- Did you enjoy sexual intercourse when you were younger? Do you still? Do you feel less sensitive or responsive during sex? If so, which parts of your body seem less sensitive?

- If you are not enjoying sex, are you experiencing pain during intercourse? Are you easily aroused or does it take you longer to become aroused? When you are aroused, does your vagina lubricate easily or has this changed?

- Have you always been orgasmic? Are you still? Have your orgasms changed? Are they less intense?

Try to be as specific as you can.

If you are unhappy because of a loss of libido, you will need to give your doctor more clues. This is intended to help you both decide if your problem is physical, emotional, relational or a mix of these. To do that, think over the following questions and be prepared to discuss any that you feel may factor into your situation.

- What else was happening in your life at the time you felt a loss of desire or libido?
- Did you experience any major life changes such as a move, a job change, children off to college, loss of a close relative?
- Do you or your partner have any serious health issues separate from the sexual side of your relationship?
- Have you or your partner experienced recent financial difficulties?
- Have either of you had an affair with another person? If yes, does your partner know about it?
- How would you characterize your relationship with your partner: Do you *both* feel you have a good marriage or partnership?
- Are there any other significant changes in your life or lifestyle that have occurred during this time?

Q: Am I alone in experiencing changes in my sexuality?

A: Hardly. A landmark 1999 study of sexual dysfunction in America, published in the *Journal of the American Medical Association* and reported in *Modern Maturity*, "pegged the rate of dysfunctional women—women who aren't interested in sex, fail to lubricate, can't reach orgasm, or experience pain—at a whopping 43 percent, versus 31 percent of men who struggle with sexual dysfunction (such as climaxing too early or failing to achieve an erection)."

Q: I am in my late 40s and recently had a hysterectomy. Since then, my libido has been nonexistent. Is this unusual? Does it happen to many women?

A: No, your loss of libido is not unusual, nor are you in a minority. After cesarean section, a hysterectomy is the most common major surgery performed on women. Nearly 20 percent of women 15 years and older have had hysterectomies and that jumps to 40 percent of women by age 60. Many have their ovaries removed at the same time, which causes a significant reduction in hormone levels, both estrogen and androgen. A large number of women (20 percent in one study) who have hysterectomies *and still have their ovaries* also have a decrease in their hormone levels. This can have a direct effect on your libido. Ask your doctor to test your hormone levels.

Q: What is a normal testosterone level?

A: The average levels of circulating testosterone in women fall between 20 and 70 nanograms per deciliter of blood. That is a wide range open to an interpretation by your doctor that will be based on a number of factors. (FYI: Men have almost twenty times as much.) For example, hormone levels fluctuate for many reasons, especially in perimenopausal women. That is one reason why your doctor will need to test your hormone levels several times and view the results in the context of your total health picture. Your physician needs to determine *what is normal for you.*

Q: When I see the doctor, what type of tests should I expect to take? How much will this cost?

A: First, you need to understand what the tests can and cannot tell your doctor. Most physicians will test your follicle stimulating hormone (FSH) level as this rises to high levels (at least 40 mIU./ml.) after menopause. Though your FSH may fluctuate widely, it indicates nothing about estrogen or testosterone. The levels do, however, provide a clue to what is happening to your hormones. Other blood tests are used to determine your testosterone picture. These include testing for total testosterone **by extraction and chromatography,** free testosterone **by equilibrium dialysis,** and sex hormone binding globulin. The methods (noted in bold type) by which these tests are performed are critical. Recognize that most commercially available blood tests for testosterone were developed for use in men, and may not be as precise when used in women, particularly menopausal women. This testing may need to be done several times in order to determine average levels. Costs vary by physician. In Simon's office, the average cost of an office visit and diagnostic tests for evaluation of libido problems is approximately $550. Insurance coverage also varies. Remember . . . many commercial labs do not perform the blood tests for testosterone in the most precise way. Your insurance company may have chosen a lab for its cost, not necessarily how it performs testosterone tests. Make sure your health care provider knows the difference. He or she can usually navigate the system if necessary. Simon's office uses the following two reference labs for these tests: Esoterix Endocrinology, 4301 Lost Hills Road, Calabasas Hills, CA 91301-5358, 800-444-9111 ext. 4045 (client services), frozen serum required. And Quest Diagnostics at Nichols Institute, 33608 Ortega

Highway, San Juan Capistrano, CA 92690-6130, 800-553-5445 (client services), www.questdiagnostics.com, frozen serum required. There may be many other qualified labs to perform these tests, and some university research centers using the methods listed above may also be good alternatives.

Q: My libido is fine, but I've noticed other physical symptoms such as memory loss, weight gain, low energy levels and free-floating anxiety. Should I be worried or get a jump-start by using testosterone?

A: This is a question for you to discuss with your doctor. If you are premenopausal, a better option is to *"jump-start" your tests*. If you can afford it, have a premenopausal hormone profile done every five to ten years, depending on your age when you start. This will allow you to correlate any changes in your energy level or your libido with changes in measurable levels of free and total testosterone. A record of your hormone levels in your prime versus changes that occur as you age will make choices much easier for you and your doctor. Remember that your hormones change dramatically from one day of the menstrual cycle to the next. Dr. Simon recommends that you use the onset of menstruation as a reasonable marker to standardize the blood testing. He recommends you have your blood drawn on menstrual cycle day 3 (the third day of menstrual flow—not spotting, staining, or anything else . . . flow). Write this day down somewhere *where you can remember it* (menstrual cycle day 3) and get your blood drawn on the same menstrual cycle day, and under the same conditions (time, lab, etc.) as possible.

Q: If I'm perimenopausal and still having periods, can I still start HRT and can I take T with it?

A: One of the more common mistakes of menopausal management is to withhold ERT/HRT from a symptomatic woman who is still menstruating. Symptoms during this time are frequent. In fact, the most common time for a woman to have hot flashes is actually *before* and not after her last period. One way to control these symptoms along with the abnormal bleeding and unintended pregnancies that commonly occur at this time is to use birth control pills. They provide both estrogen and progestogen to treat these symptoms. Oral contraceptive pills are not required, however. Lower doses of estrogen or estrogen and androgen can also be used as a supplement. For those women "in the know" this may actually seem counterintuitive. Remember that much of the perimenopausal transition is accompanied by high, not low, levels of estrogen. These high estrogen levels are what cause the increased bloating, breast tenderness, and heavy bleeding. However, once the brain becomes accustomed to these high levels any reduction in the levels leads to symptoms (i.e., hot flashes and night sweats). So you must be thinking . . . why add more estrogen? More fuel to the fire? When estrogen or estrogen and progestogen are replaced, the brain turns down its driving mechanism to the ovary, being fooled that the administered estrogen or estrogen and progestogen is actually coming from the ovaries. Once the "drive" is turned down, the ovary produces far less estrogen and a new equilibrium is established. However, the same changes that occur with ERT or HRT—that is, a reduction in free testosterone—can occur. This can lead to or aggravate libido problems. It is perfectly reasonable to add a little testosterone to the mix if this occurs.

Q: *My husband complains that I'm not as loving as I used to be. I feel fine, however. Isn't this a time in life when you're supposed to be less interested in sex?*

A: Your partner's feelings are a red flag. Does he think you are behaving differently than in the past? If so, it would be wise to ask your physician to check your hormones before your low libido is misinterpreted and your husband thinks you don't love him anymore. Because your relationship—if not your marriage—may be at risk, the effort and the expense are worth it. At least give yourself a choice.

Let's assume you have an appointment to see a physician about using estrogen-testosterone therapy. Here are some recommended questions:

Q: *Do you use the same hormone therapy for all your patients?*

A: If the answer is "yes," find another physician. There is no simple dose/response curve with supplementary testosterone—it must be tailored to your individual body chemistry. Even if you do not need testosterone, your estrogen prescription should be tailored for you as well.

Q: *How will it be decided which balance is right for me?*

A: An informed physician will express the need to work with you to "mix and match" the hormone therapy best suited to all your health needs. As we enter our 50s and 60s, we often have other health issues that must be considered—high blood pressure, digestive tract problems, etc. The health care provider must consider your body in its entirety. Be prepared to compromise, but not too much. There may also be a need for some wiggle room between your symptoms and your blood tests. Shoot for perfection, but don't expect to get it!

Q: How frequently will you monitor my testosterone levels?

A: Depending on your response to the hormones, every three to six months during the first year is a likely answer. If all is going really well, you may be able to have less laboratory testing. Save the money and take off on a romantic weekend.

Q: How soon will I see side effects if I'm going to have any?

If the testosterone level is too high, you will probably be aware by the end of the first three months of treatment and should discuss any changes that concern you with your doctor. These may include a modest increase in hair growth and a feeling of being oversexed, aroused all the time or just too sensitive in the clitoral area. However, you may also feel an increase in your energy level and sense of well-being. Part of the "mix and match" is finding the right balance. If, after three months, you do not notice any improvement, you may want to increase the amount of testosterone.

Q; What can I do to help figure out the right balance of hormones for me?

A: The single most important thing you can do is to comply with the recommended dosage on a regular basis. When hormone therapy fails, it is often because a woman does not follow instructions or the treatment may be right but the problem may be wrong. You can't treat major depression with testosterone! You can't correct a bad relationship with hormones!

Q: How long can I take testosterone?

A: The long-term effects of testosterone treatment are not completely known. The concern with oral testosterone therapy has been related to its effects on the liver. Three years of oral testosterone treatment is known to be safe while the consequences of longer treatment are not known. This is one reason why it is crucial to stay current with new information. Nonoral treatments, like patches, pellets, etc., if at physiologic levels should be safe for very long times. Remember, the ovary supplies testosterone to the body "nonorally" for a woman's entire lifetime up to and including the first few years of menopause.

Q: If I am premenopausal but am experiencing low libido, can I take testosterone?

A: Possibly. But first, your doctor should check the birth control pills you may be taking. These can have an effect on libido—and a change could make a difference. If that's not the source of the problem, the next step is to test your testosterone levels. Occasionally, but rarely, a menstruating woman will have low testosterone or free testosterone.

If you are not comfortable with the answers to these or any of your other questions during your visit with the doctor, then we encourage you to see another, better informed, physician.

Q: What do other health experts say about testosterone?

A: Your physician is most likely to refer you to a therapist in order to determine if your problem is solely hormonal or if there are emotional and relationship issues involved. For that reason, we thought it would be appropriate to have the opinions of two professionals involved with couple's therapy.

Practicing in Arlington, Virginia, Victoria Young, M.S.W., L.C.S.W., is a psychotherapist who has referred several patients to Dr. Simon. Even though, as a therapist, her focus is on treating the emotional issues in a relationship, she is alert to the physiological aspects that may be affecting a couple. "Many people have a fairly good sense of what's wrong," she said. "I encourage couples to have confidence in their own sense of things. If you have a good marriage or relationship but sexual function is a problem—and if you both feel confident that this is where the difficulty lies—work on finding a physician who specializes in this area. I encourage women to see a gynecologist who specializes in endocrinology and knows about sexuality. And for the man in the relationship, he may need to see a urologist, someone who specializes in the physiology of impotence."

Charles Michels, M.S.W., B.C.D., is a clinical social worker and therapist with Wisconsin's Marshfield Clinic. For over twenty years he has counseled men and women, particularly women, dealing with sexual dysfunction. Working in tandem with gynecologists, ob/gyns and other medical experts, he has been hearing about the new testosterone options, including the transdermal testosterone patch reviewed in Chapter Seven. As a therapist who is very familiar with all the options available to women experiencing sexual dysfunction, he is in favor of testosterone. "We need to change something around when there are clear indications that having the desire to have sex and being able to function sexually are not congruent. Something must be missing. If it were hormonal issues at play here, then it would be ridiculous not to try hormone replacement therapy—whether for sexual function, for depression or for good bone density. If testosterone can be taken safely—and it sounds to me like the transdermal patch is the safest way to take testosterone—what do you have to lose? See if it works for you."

Michels does not see testosterone as the only answer, however. He encourages a couple in a situation where a physical problem may have taken its toll on the relationship to embrace both—explore hormone replacement therapy and continue with marital counseling. "It will speed things up."

Q: What resources can I use to stay abreast of the latest research on testosterone?

A: The sources we mentioned earlier in this section for use in locating physicians are also excellent for updates on testosterone. These are:

1. The North American Menopause Society (NAMS):
   Web site: www.menopause.org and
   e-mail: info@menopause.org

2. The National Library of Medicine: Call 1-888-FIND
   NLM or go to www.nlm.nih.gov. Once there, you can
   search by subject matter.

3. The medical journal database, Medline at
   www.medlineplus.gov.

Recommended Reading

Many excellent books have been written on menopause, but their information on testosterone is sketchy or out of date. For that reason, we are recommending two, recently published, that offer good information on estrogen, testosterone and androgens in general. Additional reading—books, articles and research papers—will be found in the list of references following this chapter.

Woman: An Intimate Geography by Natalie Angier (Anchor Books, 2000). Angier's book is a well-written, insightful book that explains and explores the female body and how it works—from organs to orgasm. It has a particularly detailed and easy-to-understand description of hormones and what is known to date about their effects on the female physiology.

Sex on the Brain: The Biological Differences Between Men and Women by Deborah Blum (Viking Penguin, 1998). Blum explores the science of hormones and how they affect the brain in a clear and absorbing text.

The following information was prepared by Dr. James A. Simon for the Women's Health Research Center Web site.

Can you tell me exactly what menopause is?

Menopause is a term used to denote the point at which a woman has her last menstrual period and marks the end of a woman's reproductive years. Menopause can be brought on either as a part of the normal aging process or as a result of surgical treatment, radiation or medical therapies on both ovaries. The term *menopause* itself refers to the end of fertility as a single event. However, natural menopause rarely occurs as a sudden loss of ovarian function, but rather involves a period of waning ovarian function. This period of time that precedes the last menstrual period and up to one year following it is referred to as the peri-

157

menopausal period and represents the transition from the reproductive to the nonreproductive years. Menopause is considered "complete" when a woman has not had a menstrual period for one full year.

When does menopause occur?

At around age 45, women typically enter the perimenopausal period where they begin to experience symptoms associated with menopause. This transition period usually lasts for several years with the last physiologic event, known as menopause, occurring between ages 45 and 55 years. The average age of menopause in Western society is about 51 years with ninety-five percent of females experiencing menopause by age 55.

Besides a change in menstrual cycle, what are the other early symptoms of menopause?

The onset of menopausal symptoms varies from woman to woman to the extent that some women will experience severe multiple symptoms while other women will have few symptoms or perhaps no symptoms at all. The symptoms generally include vasomotor instability (hot flashes or hot flushes), psychological symptoms (anxiety, mood changes), and atrophic changes (thinning of soft tissues of the vagina). The most common symptom, the "hot flash" or "hot flush," occurs in approximately 80 percent of women as a result of the decrease in ovarian hormones. Hot flushes have a rapid onset and resolution and are marked by feelings of intense heat over the trunk and face, with flushing of the skin and sweating. Other symptoms that may be present include:

fatigue, nervousness, sweating, headache, insomnia, depression, irritability, joint and muscle pain, dizziness, and palpitations. The experience of going through menopause varies greatly for individual women, and women experience different symptoms to different degrees.

I'm 48 and haven't had a period in three months. I have no other symptoms. Am I in menopause? Should I see a doctor?

Menopause is defined as the last natural or "ovary-induced" menstrual period. However, menopause is not considered to be complete until a woman has not had a period for one full year. It is important that women who have missed a period see their doctor and learn what is happening. If menopause seems likely, a simple blood test to determine either the amount of follicle stimulating hormone (FSH) or the serum estradiol (E_2) concentration will help confirm whether a woman is menopausal.

What is premature menopause?

Although the average age that women reach menopause is around 50 years, there are women who enter menopause as early as age 41 or as late as age 60. When menopause occurs before the age of 40, women are considered to have entered menopause "prematurely." Premature menopause can occur as part of a woman's natural aging process, as a result of surgical removal of the ovaries because of disease such as ovarian cancer or endometriosis, or after treatment with certain medications or radiation.

Should premature menopause always be treated?

Premature menopause becomes a source of problems for most of the women who experience it. Not only does premature menopause shorten a woman's childbearing years (an important issue for those women who have waited to start a family), but it also causes an earlier onset of the consequences of aging associated with menopause, including loss of bone density, increased risk of cardiovascular disease, and deterioration of the urogenital tract. Most physicians believe that premature menopause should be treated with hormone replacement therapy to help reduce these and other risks associated with early loss of estrogen.

Is there anything you can do in your 20s and 30s to prepare for and possibly reduce these negative menopausal symptoms?

Gathering information about menopause and about the changes that occur at menopause can help prepare a woman for the transition. Though there are no guarantees, research studies have shown that there are preventative measures that women can take in their younger years that help protect them from symptoms later in life. Some modest changes in lifestyle during the 20s and 30s can have an important impact on a woman's chance of getting osteoporosis. In the early 1990s researchers were able to definitely establish that women add bone mass long after adolescence with peak mass usually being reached in a woman's early 30s. While both a woman's diet and the type and amount of exercise she is doing are two areas that affect bone strength, a woman's intake of calcium appears to have the greatest influence. A diet that includes calcium-rich foods and exercise that includes weight-bearing activity can increase peak bone mass. Other lifestyle changes that could reduce menopausal symptoms include refraining from smoking and limiting the amount of caffeine, alcohol and soda intake. Smoking has many bad consequences on a person's health, but for women, smoking also acts on the ovaries to cause earlier menopause and more years of decreased estrogen.

What exactly is a hot flash?

Hot flashes are vasomotor symptoms that are brought on when there is a rapid decline in the amount of estrogen in the body. When estrogen levels are low, an area of the brain called the hypothalamus is induced to secrete increasing amounts of gonadotropin-releasing hormone into the circulation. It is believed that the mechanism responsible for stimulating the hypothalamus also triggers the hot flashes by affecting the adjacent temperature-regulating area of the brain. Hot flashes have a rapid onset and resolution. When a hot flash occurs, a woman gets feelings of intense heat over the trunk and face, flushing of the skin, and sweating. Hot flashes may occur at night causing "night sweats," disrupted sleep patterns and insomnia. For some women the night sweats are so profound that bed linens and nightclothes need to be changed before returning to bed.

Is an increase in facial hair expected after menopause? Is it normal to be losing hair on my head, arms, legs and pubic area?

Women produce many different sex hormones, including both estrogens, commonly referred to as the "female hormones," and androgens, the "male hormones." The skin contains both estrogen receptors and androgen receptors and is, therefore, affected by changes in both hormone levels. The relative amounts of estrogen and androgen circulating in the body seem to control much of the growth or loss of body hair. If the hormone balance is disturbed, either by a decrease in estrogen at menopause or an increase in androgen, then the new balance may lead to excess androgen-related symptoms and noticeable changes in body hair distribution. Even a relative excess of androgen can lead to a male pattern of hair distribution, with hair growth occurring on the upper lip, chin and cheeks as well as a decrease in pubic, axillary and scalp hair. This situation can occur when there is an increased androgen-estrogen ratio as estrogen levels drop to a greater degree than androgens, leaving a relative androgen excess in postmenopausal women.

If a woman is using birth control pills for contraception, how will she know if she is going through menopause?

Currently, no universal criteria are available to provide a definitive answer to this question. Many physicians will simply suggest that a woman consider switching to another form of birth control after the age of 45. However, other clinicians believe that a woman who is doing well on birth control pills can continue to use the pills into her 50s. For women who continue with combined oral contraceptive pills, some may notice symptoms of menopause, such as hot flashes, during the fourth week (the pill-free week) of their cycle. Other women may not experience any symptoms. Whether symptoms are present or not, for women who are on pills and would like to know if they are entering menopause, some clinicians will obtain a serum follicle-stimulating hormone (FSH) level on day six or seven of the pill-free week. If the value is 20 IU/L or higher, the woman is switched to hormone replacement therapy at the end of the pill-free week. If the FSH is not over 20 IU/L, then birth control is continued and FSH is measured at the woman's next annual visit. However, there are some data that indicate a measure of FSH on day seven of the pill-free week may not be a sensitive enough test to determine menopause. Some clinicians do not feel comfortable relying on the results and choose to leave their patients on birth control until the patient is into her 50s. The important point to remember is that women should discuss the matter with their doctor and decide on a plan that is right for them.

What urinary symptoms are most commonly associated with menopause?

The urinary tract and the genital system develop from a common tissue source during the fetal period. Both systems are estrogen-dependent and subject to changes with menopause and a decrease in estrogen. The distal urinary tract, which includes the urethra and entrance to the bladder, atrophies as part of the general aging process, causing problems with incontinence, increased frequency of voiding, and excessive urination at night (nocturia). However, estrogen decline at menopause is thought to be an additional factor that causes more problems with bladder function for women.

What can cause depression at menopause and what can be done about it?

Psychological complaints, such as depression, may increase in menopause, but the symptoms are not specific to menopause as they also occur in other age groups albeit at a lower rate. Estrogens have been shown to play an important role in emotions as they influence the activity of central nervous system (CNS) neurotransmitters, especially the neurotransmitter serotonin known particularly for its effect on mood. Declining estrogen levels seem to reduce the availability of neurotransmitters at critical nerve sites, which may have a negative effect on emotional well-being. However, other causes unrelated to a reduction in neurotransmitter activity should also be considered. In a woman with disturbed sleep patterns secondary to hot flushes, the fatigue caused by interrupted sleep may itself cause a woman to feel depressed. Hormone replacement therapy may help reduce the hot flashes, enable a woman to sleep better, and help relieve the feelings of minor depression caused by sleep deprivation. However, hormone replacement is likely to have little or no effect on relieving depression that was brought on by other life events.

Is memory affected by menopause?

While a number of women going through menopause report problems with concentration and short-term memory, memory changes themselves have not been carefully studied in menopausal women. At present it is unclear if menopause has a direct effect on a woman's memory or if perhaps other symptoms such as mood changes, anxiety, irritability or insomnia are contributing to the perception that memory is deteriorating.

How long do menopausal symptoms last?

Vasomotor symptoms (hot flush, night sweats, palpitations, etc.) usually start about two years before menopause and continue for more than a year in at least 80 percent of affected women. For some women, symptoms will decrease in frequency and intensity within a few years, but for at least 25 percent of women, symptoms continue for more than five years. Women who choose to take hormone replacement therapy may not experience any symptoms while on therapy but may experience a return of symptoms once therapy is stopped.

How does surgical menopause differ from natural menopause?

Surgical menopause results when a woman has a bilateral oophorectomy (removal of both ovaries) with or without a hysterectomy (removal of the uterus). Surgical menopause creates a situation where the primary source of a woman's hormones is abruptly removed. When a woman goes through natural menopause, the ovaries gradually reduce production of eggs and there is associated decline in female hormones, estrogen and progesterone. This gradual regression usually occurs over the span of several years with a more dramatic reduction following the last period.

After a hysterectomy and oophorectomy, what can I expect in terms of menopausal symptoms?

Menopause brought on surgically results in an abrupt loss of the hormones produced by the ovaries, particularly estrogen. In a woman who is sensitive to estrogen's effects, the loss may cause immediate menopausal symptoms unless estrogen replacement therapy is initiated. In women who are already menopausal, the loss of ovaries may cause some further loss of estrogen but the reduction in estrogen may not be enough to produce any additional symptoms.

I had a hysterectomy years ago, but retained my ovaries. If I take hormone replacement therapy in menopause, do I need to take both estrogen and progestin?

Women who have had a hysterectomy do not need progesterone. Progesterone is given in combination with estrogen therapy as a means of protecting women from endometrial cancer caused by proliferation of the endometrium in women who receive long-term estrogen alone. For a woman without a uterus this is not a concern.

What is estrogen and where does it come from?

Estrogen is one of many steroid hormones produced in the body. Steroid hormones are produced in specific endocrine cells and then secreted into the bloodstream. The hormones travel to different sites in the body where they exert their effects. Estrogen is frequently referred to as the "female" hormone though this distinction is not completely accurate as estrogen is also produced in males just as testosterone, the "male" hormone, is produced in females. In nonpregnant women, there are three natural estrogens, frequently abbreviated as E1, E2, and E3. Estradiol (E2), the most potent human estrogen, is synthesized from testosterone and is the most important estrogen in hormone replacement therapy. The other two estrogens, estrone (E1) and estriol (E3), while present in both pre- and postmenopausal women, are less relevant since they are much weaker hormones and are commonly converted to estradiol or excreted from the body.

Estrogens used for hormone replacement therapy (HRT) come

from both natural and synthetic sources. *Natural* meaning compounds found in nature that are chemically identical to the estrogens in the human body, and *synthetic* meaning chemical compounds that do not occur in nature but are artificially synthesized to match human estrogens. Few natural sources for hormones are available. In the case of estrogen, however, a mixture can be obtained from pregnant mares' urine and is sold under the brand name Premarin (PREgnant MARe's urINe). This natural source has been used safely for HRT since the mid-1940's. Synthetic forms of estrogen are also limited to a small number of sources. All hormone replacement therapies, except for Premarin, come from three "natural" plant sources: soybeans, Chinese cactus needles, and Mexican yams. Each of these sources produces a natural product that can be transformed into hormones and used by the body.

Because the principal goal of HRT is to, as closely as possible, mimic physiologic hormone levels, estrogens that are produced in women would appear to be the best choice for treatment. However, there are some problems with using natural estrogens. Most naturally occurring estrogens (E1, E2, E3) are rapidly metabolized and excreted (with minimal effects) when administered orally. Therefore, they may be modified to improve absorption and biological efficacy. These modifications include micronization to make the particles smaller or changing the structure to resist metabolism. For example, natural estrogens are very poorly absorbed from the intestines and must be micronized before being absorbed. However, estrogens can also be manufactured synthetically or purified from natural sources with high quality and purity.

How is estrogen replacement given?

Several treatment options are available for women depending on their individual preferences. Estrogen replacement can be administered in the form of patches, pills, or creams. The advantages and disadvantages of each approach should be considered before a woman decides on the route of administration or product that is right for her.

The patch, which can be compared to wearing a Band-Aid, is applied to an area of the skin, usually on the abdomen or buttocks. Estrogen is gradually released and absorbed through the cells of the skin and moves directly into the bloodstream. Patches have to be replaced every three to seven days and care should be taken to apply them properly so the proper dose of estrogen is delivered. This method of administration allows for immediate cessation of the treatment with removal of the patch if necessary.

Oral administration is taken in much the same way as oral contraceptives, and women entering menopause may switch straight from oral contraceptive use to hormone replacement therapy. The pill is absorbed in the intestines, passes through the liver where it is metabolized and then travels through the systemic bloodstream to the tissues. Only a small fraction of the estrogen taken orally makes it past the liver's metabolism where much of the estrogen is broken down into compounds that can be excreted from the body. This process is known as the liver first-pass metabolism and results in the need for higher doses of estrogen to provide the same effects as the estrogen patch. This is one of the potential drawbacks of oral administration.

Hormone administration with creams is by vaginal delivery. The cream is applied into the vagina with a plunger in a way similar to a tampon being inserted. The cream is then absorbed through the walls of the vagina into the bloodstream and into the vaginal tissues. Since standing or moving around may cause the cream to leak out of the vagina, the cream is applied at bedtime. Some women find this method of administration "messy" and inconvenient as sexual intercourse is to be avoided immediately after the application since the cream can be absorbed through the penis into the man's body. Although many women believe that estrogen cream only affects the vaginal tissue where it is applied, in fact, estrogen administered this way is absorbed into the systemic circulation. Other vaginal delivery systems (vaginal tablet, rings, silicone rubber) for estrogen allow for lower amount of absorption.

Does estrogen replacement therapy decrease a woman's risk of developing cardiovascular problems?

Substantial evidence exists to support the protective effects of estrogen against cardiovascular disease (CVD). Epidemiological studies show that estrogen replacement therapy (ERT) significantly reduces cardiac events, like heart attacks, and cardiac mortality. The most frequent cause of CVD is atherosclerosis, a degenerative disease of the wall and inner surface of the arteries. Angiographic studies have shown that women using ERT have 50 percent to 60 percent less severe coronary stenosis than do other women even after taking into account other CVD risk factors. Additionally, for women who already suffer from coronary disease, some studies have found that ERT reduces mortality by 80 percent. The evidence gathered from research on the protective effects against heart disease of estrogens is so convincing that menopausal women who have a past history of myocardial infarction, suffer from angina or have cardiac risk factors such as diabetes, hypertension, cigarette smoking and/or an abnormal cholesterol profile should seriously consider use of ERT. For healthy women at low risk for CVD, ERT use can lower disease by 40 percent to 50 percent compared to healthy nonusers. However, some recent studies have failed to confirm these benefits, and it will be several years before the final word ("the truth") on this subject is likely to be known. By 2005, results from several large and important clinical studies will be available providing better information on the effects of estrogens on CVD.

Is there a time after which the parts of my body (heart, bones, bladder, vagina) no longer need HRT?

There are varying opinions on this topic. Some clinicians believe that hormone replacement therapy (HRT) should be administered in the smallest amount that effectively alleviates symptoms and that therapy should be limited to the shortest amount of time. For women who are using HRT to control symptoms such as hot flashes and night sweats, HRT could probably be discontinued after about two years. If these symptoms persist beyond two years in a patient who would like to discontinue HRT, the patient should try discontinuing therapy every one to three years to determine if the symptoms are still present. However, for women who are at high risk for cardiovascular disease or osteoporosis, HRT can be continued indefinitely as long as no contraindications arise.

I am on hormone replacement therapy. How often should I see my physician?

Women who are on hormone replacement therapy should see their physician at least once a year and many physicians prefer to see their patients twice a year, particularly during the first year or two after initiating treatment. More frequent visits during this time are often necessary as dosages frequently need adjustment and side effects are most likely to emerge. Additionally, a woman should contact her physician if she has any changes in symptoms or experiences abnormal vaginal bleeding between visits.

Can a menopausal woman on hormone replacement therapy become pregnant?

Women who are truly "menopausal" do not have to worry about becoming pregnant while on hormone replacement therapy (HRT) as their ovaries have stopped producing eggs. Some regimens of HRT result in regular "menstrual-like" cycles that can be confusing. These are not fertile cycles since no eggs are being released. However, for women who are still in the perimenopausal period, physicians caution patients that there is a slight chance that the ovaries may "come alive" one last time and release an egg. For this reason, women are advised to use a backup method of contraception for at least one year after their last menstrual period to avoid any surprises.

Does every woman need hormone replacement therapy (HRT)?

Each woman's symptoms and risks need to be evaluated *individually* to determine if HRT is right for them. Most physicians agree that there are three situations where HRT use should be strongly encouraged: 1) women with induced surgical menopause (removal of both the ovaries in the premenopausal years), which results in an abrupt interruption of endogenous estrogen production and acute onset of symptoms such as hot flushes and night sweats; 2) women with severe symptoms of estrogen deficiency during perimenopause and menopause; and 3) women who have a spontaneous, albeit premature menopause, particularly if before the age of 40 years old or even 45 years old. For women who are not affected by any of these three conditions, some seem to continue to make enough estrogen on their own to compensate for the ovaries' cessation of estrogen production. For women who have no symptoms of estrogen deprivation and for women whose risk of cardiovascular disease and osteoporosis can be managed using nonhormonal medications, hormone replacement therapy might not be right for them. However, estrogen replacement is recommended for the following groups of women, as it can reduce long-term health risks: 1) women with a family history and/or personal history that is consistent with a high risk of CVD; 2) women with a family history and/or personal history that is consistent with a high risk of osteoporosis; and 3) women with premature menopause (at or before age 40) as such an early loss of estrogen puts them at particularly high risk for both CVD and osteoporosis. Women who have received or are receiving treatment for breast cancer or high-grade uterine cancers should not take hormone replacement except under very special circumstances.

Can I take HRT if I have a benign fibroid tumor in my breast or uterus?

Until recently, many physicians have advised women with either of these conditions that HRT was probably not the right choice for them. However, with the low dose of estrogen used today in replacement therapy, the answer to this question is no longer a definite no and should not deter women from using HRT. However, women with fibroid tumors will need to work closely with their physicians to ensure that the fibroid is not growing and, even if the size is increasing, to determine if HRT is the cause or whether there is another contributing factor. Also, some women with fibroid tumors of the uterus experience irregular or heavy bleeding when on HRT and choose not to continue with treatment. The positive benefits of HRT on maintaining strong bones and a higher quality of life need to be weighed against the worry associated with benign tumors. The best approach is for a woman to discuss the issue with her physician.

What can I do about the amount of weight I've gained since beginning ERT?

Estrogen does not cause weight gain. In fact, estrogen actually works to decrease abdominal obesity. Menopause itself, which comes at a time when a woman's metabolism is slowing down, is more likely the cause of any increase in weight. Yet, despite the lack of evidence to support the idea that ERT increases weight, some women insist that it increases their appetite. While about 25 percent of women who start ERT report a slight weight gain, the exact cause of the increase is not clear but appears to be unrelated to ERT.

Does hormone replacement therapy cause menstrual periods to continue? For how long? Will I go on menstruating forever?

In the past, clinicians tended to inform women that they shouldn't expect much bleeding while on hormone replacement therapy (HRT), and as a result, women have been surprised when they continue to experience bleeding. While some women like to continue to have monthly bleeding cycles, many women look forward to the time in their lives when they no longer have periods. Women who choose HRT are most likely going to experience some amount of bleeding. How much or when the bleeding occurs, however, depends in part on the type of HRT regimen chosen. Women who choose to use continuous estrogen/progestin regimens tend to stop bleeding within four to six months and the bleeding they do experience is usually very light or more often just spotting or staining. Women who use cyclic HRT regimes, meaning that there are some days where only estrogen is taken and other days when both estrogen and progestin are taken, continue having withdrawal bleeding for a longer period of time. These cyclic "menstrual-like" bleeding episodes are usually predictable but may continue beyond the age of sixty. Generally, most women will achieve amenorrhea, cessation of menstrual bleeding, within the first three years of cyclic HRT use.

Is there a relationship between hormone replacement therapy and cancer?

Breast cancer is the most feared disease among women, and the assumption that hormone replacement therapy (HRT) may increase this risk is the main reason why many women refuse to use hormones. Additionally, the fear of uterine cancer was the reason that estrogen replacement therapy was withdrawn in the 1970s. Shortly after hormone therapy first became available for use over 40 years ago, the FDA put out a warning against giving hormones to women with breast cancer and benign breast disease. The studies that led to this announcement utilized higher doses of HRT and oral contraceptives than are used today.

Even though lower doses of estrogen are used today and current studies published on the association between hormone use and breast cancer have not shown a definitive relationship, many women continue to believe that HRT causes breast cancer. The fact is that many epidemiological studies have been published on the association between hormone use and breast cancer. Most of the studies indicated that use of estrogen does not increase a woman's risk of developing breast cancer. Findings from the current research has led to the following conclusions. Estrogen monotherapy (use of estrogen without progestin), for less than ten years, does not appear to significantly increase the risk of breast cancer. There is some modest evidence to suggest that long-term use of estrogen/progestin combinations (more than 10 years of use) may increase the risk of breast cancer slightly. However, this risk refers only to the number of women that get breast cancer (morbidity rate), and not to the number of women who die from breast cancer (mortality rate). If the mortality rate is considered instead of morbidity, the evidence clearly shows that women who use hormone replacement actually have a decreased risk of dying from the disease. Additionally, women using HRT usually get regular medical checks, have increased use of mammography screening, and are carefully monitored so that if breast cancer is detected, it can be treated at an earlier stage. These health practices, themselves, tend to increase the number of breast cancer cases discovered.

The relationship between uterine cancer and estrogen use is much clearer. We know that estrogens, both endogenous and exogenous, cause the endometrium to proliferate. Under prolonged estrogenic stimulation and in the absence of opposing progestogen use, the endometrial cells continue to multiply, a process known as hyperplasia. Hyperplasia is a major risk factor for endometrial cancer. However, the risk of cancer can be all but eliminated with the proper use of progestogen.

If I have a family history of breast cancer, can HRT be dangerous?
The information provided to both physicians and the public regarding the risks of HRT use in women with family history of breast cancer is confusing. Many women in this situation do not want to take hormones and many physicians do not prescribe them for their patients with a family history of the disease. A woman whose mother or sister had a breast malignancy has only a slight increase in her own risk of developing breast cancer if the relative's cancer developed after menopause. However, the risk increases more substantially (two to three times greater) if the mother's cancer began before menopause. For women with family histories of breast cancer, the decision to take HRT often comes down to quality of life issues where women have to weigh their menopausal symptoms against the risks.

I have had breast cancer. Can I take HRT?
Some authorities consider existing or recently treated cancer of the breast to be an absolute contraindication, while others do not

believe that HRT is an absolute contraindication and can be given in certain cases if the patient receives close medical surveillance. While studies on HRT in women who have had breast cancer do not confirm an increased risk of recurrence, other medications (e.g., Tamoxifen), may actually reduce a woman's risk of a recurrence of breast cancer. Unfortunately, these agents (e.g., Tamoxifen) may increase menopausal symptoms and cannot be used with HRT.

What is osteoporosis?

Osteoporosis is a common bone disease that affects both men and women. The disease is characterized by a loss of bone mass as the bone begins to disintegrate and become more porous. As the bones become more porous, fractures begin to occur even without trauma, and bone fractures make osteoporosis a major medical concern. In fact, almost all bone fractures that occur in postmenopausal women and elderly men are osteoporotic fractures resulting from bone that has become thin and weak. For some women with osteoporosis of the spine, even a hug can cause a spine fracture.

Why are so many women afflicted with osteoporosis?

Among white women living to 80 years of age, about one-third will suffer at least one hip fracture and many will have two. White women who live to this age have almost a 50 percent chance of suffering an osteoporotic fracture of the spine, hip or forearm. It is important to remember that bones are living tissue that are constantly being remodeled and repaired, and estrogen status plays a critical role in achieving and maintaining bone mass. Estrogen also plays an important role in bone metabolism by influencing the exchange of calcium with the blood. There are three ways in which estrogen acts: 1) by facilitating the uptake of calcium from food; 2) by improving the movement of calcium from the blood into the bone; and 3) by inhibiting the loss of calcium from the bone.

Males and females build bone mass until they reach about 30 years old. After this point, bone will be lost at a slow rate of about one percent a year. However, at menopause, the drop in estrogen levels accelerates the deterioration of bone tissue to about three percent per year for seven to ten years before slowing down again. So if a woman is menopausal at age 50, without estrogen supplements, by the time she is age 60, she could have lost up to 30 percent of her bone mass.

What causes the difference in bone loss between women and men?

Osteoporosis in men has received much less attention, not because men are not affected by the disease, rather it seems that men have been ignored in early studies since fractures in men tend to occur at least ten to 15 years later than in women. There are several factors that influence this later onset: 1) men achieve a higher peak bone mass in their 30s than women do and thus have more mass to lose before the risk of fracture is high; 2) men's bones have a greater cross-sectional area and are larger in size; and 3) aging men do not experience the period of accelerated bone loss associated with menopause.

How do I know if I am at risk for osteoporosis?

Osteoporosis is associated with many different risk factors. Some of these risk factors can be modified and some cannot. Risk factors that cannot be modified include: family history of osteoporosis; personal history of a fracture as an adult; Caucasian race; advanced age; female gender; early menopause; small, thin stature; and poor health or frailty. The potential factors that can be modified include: current cigarette smoking, low body weight, estrogen deficiency, low calcium intake, alcoholism, taking medications that decrease calcium and inadequate physical exercise.

How much risk is hereditary?

Heredity is considered a major risk factor for the development of osteoporosis, and there is clear evidence to support this view. Each person inherits a genetic tendency that will determine to a certain extent the size and strength of their bones. Individuals who have blond or red hair, fair skin, freckles, the propensity to bruise, a small frame, and adolescent scoliosis are considered to have a genetic predisposition to have osteoporosis develop.

What can I do to prevent osteoporosis?

Individuals can work toward modifying their risk for osteoporosis through maintaining good health and adopting lifestyle habits that maximize bone development and minimize bone loss. Ideally, these habits should be established early in life, at least by the teen years, and continue throughout a person's lifetime. However, no matter what a person's age, it is never too late to make changes that can help prevent osteoporosis. Eating calcium-rich foods, performing weight-bearing exercises, abstaining from smoking, and limiting alcohol, caffeine and soda intake will help bones stay stronger. Additionally, for women who are menopausal, estrogen replacement therapy can slow the acceleration of bone loss that begins at menopause. While many women are hesitant to use hormone replacement, it is important to note that there are now several other agents proven to prevent osteoporosis. These include estrogen receptor modulators (SERMs) like raloxifene HCI (Evista from Eli Lilly) and the bisphosphonates, alendronate (Fosamax from Merck) and risedronate (Actonel from Proctor & Gamble).

I have many of the risk factors for osteoporosis. What should I do?

Discussing osteoporosis with your physician is important. Before making a diagnosis of osteoporosis, your doctor should complete a medical history and thorough physical examination. While there is some debate in the medical community and certainly among insurance companies, many physicians believe that women should also have a baseline bone-density scan when they enter menopause so that treatment can be monitored and adjusted as needed.

Does estrogen replacement therapy help to prevent postmenopausal osteoporosis?

Estrogen has been the most studied and the most used agent for prevention of osteoporosis. If used in appropriate doses, hormone therapy will almost always prevent the disease, providing that calcium levels are adequate as well. The goal of bone treatment involves balancing bone formation with bone resorption (breakdown). Estrogen greatly reduces bone loss incurred at menopause that stems from estrogen deficiency by maintaining mineral strength and mass. Estrogens, SERMs, and bisphosphonates have all been proven to work better than placebos or calcium alone.

If I want to use hormone replacement therapy or one of the other agents to prevent osteoporosis, how long would I have to continue to take these drugs?

Since the average age of menopause is 51 years and generally most women will not incur a fracture until her 70s, many women are left wondering if, by stopping their hormone therapy or other bone sparing medications, they will lose the benefits they gained while on it. The answer is both yes and no. Women who start osteoporosis prevention therapy at menopause and continue it for seven to ten years gain long-term protection against osteoporotic fractures. Most studies show that bone that has been maintained while on treatment will not be lost immediately when treatment stops. However, bone loss recurs at the same rapid rate as before treatment, so by seven to ten years later there would be no net benefit.

So the question remains, how long should women stay on osteoporosis prevention therapy? The fact is there is no easy answer. Since each woman's risks and personal history varies, there is no one recommendation appropriate for all. Many studies suggest that osteoporosis prevention therapy should be a lifelong therapy. However, currently ten years of treatment is considered optimal to protect against bone loss and prevent fractures with more research needed before longer treatments can be safely recommended. In the meantime, women should review their own situation with their physician before making a decision whether to continue treatment or stop.

Adams, M. R., J. K. Williams, J. R. Kaplan, "Effects of androgens on coronary artery atherosclerosis and atherosclerosis-related impairment of vascular responsiveness." *Arterioscler. Thromb. Vasc. Biol.* 1995; 15:562–570.

Adashi, E. "The climacteric ovary as a functional gonadotropin-driven androgen producing gland." *Fertil Steril.* 1994; 62:20–27.

Albertazzi, P., R. Di Micco, E. Zanardi, "Tibolone: a review." *Maturitas.* 1998; 30:295–305.

Almeida, O. P. "Sex playing with the mind. Effects of estrogen and testosterone on mood and cognition." *Arq Neuropsiquiatr* 1999 Sep; 57(3A): 701–6.

Aloia, J. F., A. Kapoor, A. Vaswani, S. H. Cohen, "Changes in body composition following therapy of osteoporosis with methandrostenolone." *Metabolism.* 1981; 30:1076–1079.

Altman, Alan M., and Laurie Ashner. *Making Love the Way We Used To . . . Or Better.* Chicago: Contemporary Books, 2001.

Angier, Natalie. *Woman, An Intimate Geography.* New York: Anchor Books, 2000.

Bancroft, J. "Endocrinology of Sexual Function." *Clinics in Obstetrics and Gynecology* 7(2) (1980): 253–281.

Bancroft, J., et al. "Androgens and Sexual Behavior in Women Using Oral Contraceptives." *Clinical Endocrinology* 12 (1980): 327–340.

Barrett-Connor E., D. Goodman-Gruen, "Prospective study of endogenous sex hormones and fatal cardiovascular disease in postmenopausal women." *BMJ.* 1995; 311:1193–1196.

Barrett-Connor, E., C. Timmons, R. Young, et al. "Interim safety analysis of a two-year study comparing oral estrogen-androgen and conjugated estrogens in surgically menopausal women." *Journal of Women's Health* 1996; 5, 593–602.

Barrett-Connor, E., R. Young, M. Notelovitz, et al. "A two-year, double-blind comparison of estrogen-androgen and conjugated estrogens in surgically menopausal women. Effects on bone mineral density, symptoms and lipid profiles." *J. Reprod. Med.* 1999; 44:1012–1020.

Basson, Rosemary. "The Female Sexual Response: A Different Model." *Journal of Sex & Marital Therapy*, 26:51–65, 2000.

Basson, R., J. Berman, A. Burnett, L. Derogatis, D. Ferguson, J. Fourcroy, I. Goldstein, A. Graziottin, J. Heiman, E. Laan, S. Leiblum, H. Padma-Nathan, R. Rosen, K. Segraves, R. T. Segraves, R. Shabsigh, M. Sipski, G. Wagner, B. Whipple, "Report of the International Consensus Development Conference on Female Sexual Dysfunction: Definitions and Classifications." *The Journal of Urology.* 2000; 163:888–893.

Beck, J. "Hypoactive Sexual Desire Disorder: An Overview." *Jour-*

nal of Consulting and Clinical Psychology, 63(6) (1995): 919–923.

Berrino, F., P. Muti, A. Micheli, et al. "Serum sex hormone levels after menopause and subsequent breast cancer." *J. Natl. Cancer Inst.* 1996; 88:291–296.

Birrell, S. N., J. M. Bentel, T. E. Hickey, et al. "Androgens induce divergent proliferative responses in human breast cancer cell lines." *J. Steroid Biochem. Molec. Biol.* 1995; 52; 459–467.

Bixo, M., T. Backstrom, B. Winblad, A. Andersson, "Estradiol and testosterone in specific regions of the human female brain in different endocrine states." *J. Steroid Biochem. Mol. Biol.* 1995; 55:297–303.

Blum, Deborah. *Sex on the Brain.* New York: Penguin Group, 1998.

Botsis, D., D. Kassanos, D. Kalogirou, G. Antoniou, N. Vitoratos, P. Karakitsos, "Vaginal ultrasound of the endometrium in post-menopausal women with symptoms of urogenital atrophy on low-dose estrogen or tibolone treatment: a comparison." *Maturitas.* 1977; 26:57–62.

Boulet, M. F., B. J. Oddens, "Female voice changes around and after the menopause—an initial investigation." *Maturitas.* 1996; 23:15–21.

Brinbeg, C. H., R. Kurzrok, "Low-dosage androgen-estrogen therapy in the older age group. Symposium presentation." *J. Am. Geriatr. Soc.* 1955; 3:656-666.

Brody, Jane. "A Tad of Testosterone Adds Zest to Menopause," *The New York Times* (February 24, 1998).

Buckler, H. M., W. R. Robertson, "Which Androgen Replacement Therapy for Women?" *Journal of Clinical Endocrinology and Metabolism.* 1998; Nov; 83(11):3920–3924.

Burger, H. G., J. Hailes, M. Menelaus, J. Nelson, et al. "The management of persistent menopausal symptoms with oestradioltestosterone implants: clinical, lipid and hormonal results." *Maturitas*. 1984; 6:351–358.

Castelo-Branco, C., E. Ccasals, F. Figueras, et al. "Two-year prospective and comparative study on the effects of tibolone on lipid pattern, behavior of apolipoproteins Al and B." *Menopause*. 1999; 6:92–97.

Davis, S. "Androgen Replacement in Women: A Commentary." *The Journal of Endocrinology & Metabolism*. 1999; 84:1886–1891.

Davis, S. R., P. I. McCloud, B. J. G. Strauss, H. G. Burger, "Testosterone enhances estradiol's effects on postmenopausal bone density and sexuality." *Maturitas*. 1995; 21:227–236.

Demers, L. "Biochemistry and Laboratory Measurement of Androgens in Women." In *Androgenic Disorders*, edited by G. P. Redmond. New York: Raven Press, Ltd., 1995, pp. 21–34.

Derogatis, L. "The Derogatis Interview for Sexual Functioning (DISF/DISF-SR): An Introductory Report." *Journal of Sex & Marital Therapy*. 1997; 23:291–304.

Derogatis, L. R., B. Conklin-Powers, "Psychological assessment measures of female sexual functioning in clinical trials." *International Journal of Impotence Research*. 1998; 10:S111–S116.

Diamond, J. *The Evolution of Human Sexuality*. New York: Basic Books, 1997.

Dobs, A. S., T. Nguyen, C. Pace, "Differential Effects of Oral Estrogen versus Oral Estrogen-Androgen Replacement Therapy on Body Composition in Postmenopausal Women." Paper in press.

Dorgan, J. F., C. Longcope, H. E. Stephenson, Jr., et al. "Relation of prediagnostic serum estrogen and androgen levels to breast cancer risk." *Cancer Epidemiol. Biomarkers Prev.* 1996; 180: S325–S327.

Drake, E. B., V. W. Henderson, F. Z. Stanczyk, C. A. McCleary,

W. S. Brown, C. A. Smith, A. A. Rizzo, G. A. Murdock, J. G. Buckwalter, "Associations between circulating sex steroid hormones and cognition in normal elderly women." *Neurology* 2000 Feb 8; 54(3):599–603.

Geist, S. H., U. J. Salmon. 1941 "Androgen therapy in gynecology." *JAMA.* 2207–2213.

Gelfand, M. M. "Role of androgens in surgical menopause." *Am. J. Obstet. Gynecol.* 1999; 180:325–327.

Gelfand, M., B. Wiita, "Androgen and estrogen-androgen hormone replacement therapy: A review of the safety literature," 1941–1996. *Clinical Therapeutics* 1997; 19, 383–404.

Gerritsma, E. J., M. P. Brocaar, M. M. Hakkesteegt, J. D. Birkenhager, "Virilization of the voice in postmenopausal women due to the anabolic steroid nandrolone decanoate." The effects of medication for one year. *Clin. Otolaryngol.* 1994; 19:79–84.

Gitlin, N., P. Korner, H. M. Yang. "Liver function in postmenopausal women on estrogen-androgen hormone replacement therapy: A meta-analysis of eight clinical trials." *Menopause* 1999; 6, 216–224.

Gorgels, W. J., Y. v d Graaf, M. A. Blankenstein, H. J. Collette, D. W. Erkelens, J. D. Banga. "Urinary sex hormone excretions in premenopausal women and coronary heart disease risk: a nested case-referent study in the DOM-cohort." *J. Clin. Epidemiol.* 1997 Mar; 50(3): 275–81.

Gouchie, C., D. Kimura, "The relationship between testosterone levels and cognitive ability patterns." *Psychoneuroendocrinology.* 1991; 16:323–334.

Graham, C., and B. Sherwin. "The Relationship between Mood and Sexuality in Women Using an Oral Contraceptive As a Treatment for Premenstrual Symptoms." *Psychoneuroimmunology* 18(4) (1993): 273–281.

Gruber, D. M., M. O. Sator, S. Kirchengast, E. A. Joura, J. C.

Huber, "Effect of percutaneous androgen replacement therapy on body composition and body weight in postmenopausal women." *Maturitas* 1998; 29:253–259.

Guo, S. S., C. Zeller, W. C. Chumlea, R. M. Siervogel, "Aging, body composition and lifestyle: the Fels Longitudinal Study." *American Journal of Clinical Nutrition* 1999; 70:405–411.

Haarbo, J., U. Marsle, A. Gotfredsen, C. Christiansen, "Postmenopausal hormone replacement therapy prevents central distribution of body fat after menopause." *Metabolism* 1991; 40: 1323–1326.

Halpern, C., J. Udry, and C. Suchindran, "Testosterone Predicts Initiation of Coitus in Adolescent Females." *Psychosomatic Medicine* 59 (1997); 161–171.

Hanggi, W., Jaeger, F., Lippuner, H. Birkhauser, F. F. Horber, "Differential impact of conventional oral or transdermal hormone replacement therapy or tibolone on body composition in postmenopausal women." *Clinical Endocrinology* 1998; 48: 691–699.

Hickok, L., C. Toomey, L. Speroff, "A comparison of esterified estrogens with and without methyltestosterone: Effects on endometrial histology and serum lipoproteins in postmenopausal women." *Obstetrics and Gynecology* 1993; 6: 919–924.

Hitt, Jack. "The Second Sexual Revolution," *The New York Times Magazine* (February 20, 2000).

Holstein, Lana, L. *How to Have Magnificent Sex.* New York: Crown Publishing Group, 2001.

Honoré, E. K., J. K. Williams, M. R. Adams, D. M. Ackerman, J. D. Wagner, "Methyltestosterone does not diminish the beneficial effects of estrogen replacement therapy on coronary artery reactivity in cynomolgus monkeys." *Menopause.* 1996; 3: 20–26.

Howe, R. S., R. P. Chow, C. L. Stevens, "Use of flutamide for self-induced androgen excess: a case report." *J, Reprod. Med.* 1994; 39:838–840.

Jassal, S. K., E. Barrett-Connor, S. L. Edelstein, "Low bioavailable testosterone levels predict future height loss in postmenopausal women." *J. Bone Mineral Res.* 1995; 10:650–654.

Judd, H. L., N. Fournet, "Changes in ovarian hormone function with aging." *Exp. Gerontol.* 1994; 29:285–298.

Kaplan, H. S., *The New Sex Therapy*. New York: Brunner/Mazer, 1974.

Kaplan, H. S., T. Owett, "The female androgen deficiency syndrome." *J. Sex Marital Ther.* 1993; 19:3–24.

Kay, G. G., J. A. Simon, T. Huh, M. Shepanek, A. Artis, B. Wiita, "Cognitive function, mood, and quality of life: double-blind comparison of estrogen (esterified estrogens) and estrogen-androgen (esterified estrogens + methyltestosterone) therapy in surgically menopausal women." Eighth Annual Meeting of the North American Menopause Society, Boston, MA, September 16–19, 1997.

Khosla, S., J. Melton, E. J. Atkinson, et al. "Relationship of serum sex steroid levels and bone turnover markers with bone mineral density in men and women." *J. Clin. Endocrinol. Metab.* 1998; 83:2266–2274.

Labrie, F., P. Diamond, L. Cusan, et al. Effect of 12-month dehydroepiandrosterone replacement therapy on bone, vagina and endometrium in postmenopausal women. *J. Clin. Endocrinol. Metab.* 1997; 82:3498–3505.

Laughlin, G., E. Barrett-Connor, D. Kritz-Silverstein, D. von Muhlen, "Hysterectomy, Oophorectomy, and Endogenous Sex Hormone Levels in Older Women: The Rancho Bernardo Study. *The J. Clin. Endocrinol. & Metab.* 2000; 85:645–651.

Leland, John. "The Science of Women and Sex," *Newsweek* (May 29, 2000).

Lindholm, P., E. Vilkman, T. Raudaskoski, E. Suvanto-Luukkonen, A. Kauppila, "The effect of postmenopause and postmenopausal HRT on measured voice values and vocal symptoms." *Maturitas.* 1997; 28:47–53.

Longcope, C. "Hormone dynamics at the menopause." *Ann. NY Acad. Sci.* 1990; 592:21–30.

Longcope, C. "Metabolism of dehydroepiandrosterone." *Ann. NY Acad. Sci.* 1995; 774:143–148.

Longcope, C., R. S. Baker, S. L. Hui, C. C. Johnston, Jr. "Androgen and estrogen dynamics in women with vertebral crush fractures." *Maturitas.* 1984; 6:309–318.

Longcope, C., S. Baker "Androgen and estrogen dynamics: relationships with age, weight and menopause status." *J. Clin Endocrinol. Metab.* 1993; 76:601–604.

Longcope, C., C. Bourget, C. Flood, "The production and aromatization of dehydroepiandrosterone in postmenopausal women. *Maturitas.* 1982; 4:325–332.

Longcope, C., C. Franz, C. Morello, R. Baker, C. C. Johnson, Jr. "Steroid and gonadotropin levels in women during the perimenopausal years." *Maturitas.* 1986; 8:189–196.

Mazer, N. "New clinical applications of transdermal testosterone delivery in men and women." *Journal of Controlled Release.* 2000 March 1; 65(1–2):303–315.

McEwen, B. "Protective and Damaging Effects of Stress Mediators." *The New England Journal of Medicine* 338(3) (1998): 171–179.

Mendel, C. M. "The free hormone hypothesis. Distinction from the free hormone transport hypothesis." *J. Androl.* 1992; 13: 107–116.

Miller, B. E., M. J. De Souza, K. Slade, A. A. Luciano, "Sublingual administration of micronized estradiol and progesterone, with and without micronized testosterone: effect on biochemical markers of bone metabolism and bone mineral density." *Menopause* 2000 Sep–Oct; 7(5): 318–26.

North American Menopause Society. Menopause Core Curriculum Study Guide.

Northrup, Christiane. *The Wisdom of Menopause: Creating Physical and Emotional Health and Healing During the Change.* New York: Bantam, 2001.

Orentreich, N., J. L. Brind, R. L. Rizer, J. H. Vogelman, "Age changes and sex differences in serum dehydroepiandrosterone sulfate concentrations throughout adulthood." *J. Clin. Endocrinol. Metab.* 1984; 59:551–555.

Phillips, E., Bauman, C. "Safety surveillance of esterified estrogens-methyltestosterone (Estratest and Estratest HS) replacement therapy in the United States." *Clin. Ther.* 1997; 19:1070–1084.

Phillips, G. B., B. H. Pinkernell, T. Y. Jing, "Relationship between serum sex hormones and coronary artery disease in postmenopausal women." *Arterioscler. Thromb. Vasc. Biol.* 1997; 17: 695–701.

Plouffe, L., J. A. Simon, "Androgen effects on the central nervous system in the postmenopausal woman." *Semin. Reprod. Endocrinol.* 1998; 16:135–143.

Potts, M., R. Short, *Ever Since Adam and Eve: The Evolution of Human Sexuality.* New York: Cambridge Press, 1999.

Rae, Stephen. "rx: desire," *Modern Maturity* (March/April 2001).

Raisz, L. G., B. Wiita, A. Artis, et al. "Comparison of the effects of estrogen alone and estrogen plus androgen on biochemical markers of bone formation and resorption in postmenopausal women. *J. of Clin. Endocrinol. and Metab.* 1996; 81:37–43.

Rako, S. *The Hormone of Desire.* New York: Harmony, 1996.

Reichman J. *I'm Not in the Mood.* New York: William Morrow and Company, 1998.

Rosen, R., C. Brown, J. Heiman, S. Leiblum, C. Meston, R. Shabsigh, D. Ferguson, R. D'Agostino, "The Female Sexual Function Inde (FSFI): A Multidimensional Self-Report Instrument for the Assessment of Female Sexual Function." *Journal of Sex & Marital Therapy.* 2000; 26:191–208.

Rosen, R., and S. Leiblum, "Hypoactive Sexual Desire." Clinical Sexuality 10(1) 1(1995): 107–121.

Rosenberg, M., R. King, and C. Timmons, "Estrogen-Androgen for Hormone Replacement: A Review." *The Journal of Reproductive Medicine* 42(7) (1997): 394–402.

Sands, R., and J. Studd, "Exogenous Androgens in Postmenopausal Women." *The American Journal of Medicine.* 98(suppl 1A) (1995): 76–79.

Sarrel, P., B. Dobay, B. Wiita, "Estrogen and estrogen-androgen replacement in postmenopausal women dissatisfied with estrogen-only therapy: Sexual behavior and neuroendocrine responses." *Journal of Reproductive Medicine* 1998; 43,847–856.

Sarrel, P. M. "Psychosexual effects of Menopause: Role of Androgens." *Am. J. Obstet. Gynecol.* 1999 March; 180 (3 Pt 2): S319–24.

Sarrel, P. M., K. L. Giblin, B. A. Block, "Sexual interest and functioning in postmenopausal women: A community based national survey." *Menopause* 1998; 5:262.

Sarrel P. M., B. Wiita, "Vasodilator effects of estrogen are not diminished by androgen in postmenopausal women." *Fertility and Sterility* 1997; 68,1125–1127.

Sayegh, R. A., L. Kelly, J. Wurtman, A. Deitch, D. Chelmow, "Impact of hormone replacement therapy on body mass and fat compositions of menopausal women: a cross-sectional study." *Menopause* 1999; 6:312–315.

Scheiner-Engel, P. et al. "Low Sexual Desire in Women: The Role of Reproductive Hormones." *Hormones and Behavior* 23 (1989): 221–234.

Sherfey, M. J. *The Nature of Evolution of Female Sexuality*. New York: Random House, 1972.

Sherwin, B. B. "Affective changes with estrogen and androgen replacement therapy in surgically menopausal women." *J. Affect. Discord.* 1988; 14:177–187.

Sherwin, B. B., M. M. Gelfand, "Differential symptom response to parenteral estrogen and/or androgen administration in the surgical menopause." *Am. J. Obstet. Gynecol.* 1985; 151:153–160.

Sherwin, B. B., M. M. Gelfand, "The role of androgen in the maintenance of sexual functioning in oophorectomized women." *Psychosom. Med.* 1987; 49:397–409.

Sherwin, B. B., T. Owett "The Female Androgen Deficiency Syndrome." *Journal of Sex & Marital Therapy.* 19(1) (1993): 3–24.

Shifren J., G. Braunstein, J. Simon, P. Casson, J. Buster, G. Redmond, R. Burki, E. Ginsburg, R. Rosen, S. Leiblum, K. Caramelli, N. Mazer, "Transdermal Testosterone Treatment in Women with Impaired Sexual Function After Oophorectomy." *The New England Journal of Medicine.* 2000:343:682–688.

Simon, J. A. "Surgically Induced Menopause." *The Female Patient.* 2001; 26:50–51.

Simon, J. A. "Understanding Perimenopause." In: *No More Hot Flashes and Even More Good News* (Budoff, P. W., ed.), New York: Warner Books, Inc., pp. 9–36, 1998.

Simon, J. A., Kay, G., Eberle, C. "Effects of Progestins and Progesterone on CNS Function." *Menopausal Medicine.* 6(4):8–12, Winter, 1998.

Simon, J. A., E. Klaiber, B. Wiita, A. Bowen, H. M. Yang, "Differential effects of estrogen-androgen and estrogen-only therapy on vasomotor symptoms, gonadotropin secretion, and endogenous androgen bioavailability in postmenopausal women." *Menopause.* 1999; 6:138–146.

Siseles, N. O., H. Halperin, H. J. Benencia, et al. "A comparative study of two hormone replacement therapy regimens on safety and efficacy variables." *Maturitas.* 1995; 21:210–210.

Slayden, S. "Risks of Menopausal Androgen Supplementation." *Seminars in Reproductive Endocrinology.* 1998; 16(2):145–152.

Studd, J. W., W. P. Colins, S. Chakravarti, "Estradiol and testosterone implants in the treatment of psychosexual problems in postmenopausal women." *Br. J. Obstet. Gynaecol.* 1977; 84: 314–315.

Sullivan, Andrew. "Why Men Are Different," *The New York Times Magazine* (April 2, 2000).

Taaffe, D. R., M. L. Villa, R. Delay, et al. "Maximal muscle strength of elderly women is not influenced by estrogen status." *Age Aging* 24; 1995; 329–333.

Tagatz, G. E., R. A. Kopher, T. C. Nagel, T. Okagaki, "The clitoral index: a bioassay of androgenic stimulation." *Obstet Gynecol.* 1979; 54:562–564.

U.S. Department of Health and Human Services. *Women: A Developmental Perspective.* National Institutes of Health: Publication #82–2298, April 1982.

U.S. Department of Health and Human Services, Food and Drug Administration, Center for Drug Evaluation and Research. *Guidance for Industry, Female Sexual Dysfunction: Clinical Development of Drug Products for Treatment.* May 2000.

Urman, B., S. M. Pride, B. H. Yuen, "Elevated serum testosterone, hirsutism, and virilism associated with combined androgenestrogen hormone replacement therapy." *Obstet. Gynecol.* 1991; 77:595–598.

Verkauf, B. S., J. Van Thron, W. F. O'Brien, "Clitoral size in normal women." *Obstet. Gynecol.* 1992; 85:529–537.

Vermeulen, A. "The hormonal activity of the postmenopausal ovary." *J. Clin. Endocrinol. Metab.* 1976; 42:247–253.

Vermeulen, A. "Sex hormone status of the postmenopausal woman." *Maturitas.* 1980; 2:81–89.

Vermeulen, A., S. Goemaere, J. M. Kaufman, "Testosterone, body composition and aging." *Journal of Endocrinological Investigation* 1999; 22:110–116.

Wagner, J., L. Zhang, K. Williams, et al. "Esterified estrogens with and without methyltestosterone decrease arterial LDL metabolism in cynomolgus monkeys." *Arteriosclerosis, Thrombosis, and Vascular Biology* 1996; 16, 1473–1480.

Wang, C., R. S. Swerdloff, A. Iranmanesh, A. Dobs, P. Snyder, G. Cunningham, et al. "Transdermal testosterone gel improves sexual function, mood, muscle strength, and body composition parameters in hypogonadal men." *J. of Clin. Endocrinol. & Metab.* 2000; 85:2839–2853.

Warnock, J. K., J. C. Bundren, D. W. Morris, "Female, hypoactive sexual desire disorder due to androgen deficiency: clinical and psychometric." *Psychopharmacol Bull.* 1997; 33:761–766.

Warnock, J. K., J. C. Bundren, D. W. Morris, "Female Hypoactive Sexual Disorder: Case Studies of Physiologic Androgen Replacement." *Journal of Sex & Marital Therapy.* 1999 Jul–Sep; 25(3): 175–182.

Watts, N. B., M. Notelovitz, M. C. Timmons W. A. Addison, B. Wiita, L. J. Downey, "Comparison of oral estrogens and estrogens plus androgen on bone mineral density, menopausal symptoms, and lipid-lipoprotein profiles in surgical menopause." *Obstetrics & Gynecology.* 1995; 85:529–537.

Wimalawansa, S. J. "Prevention and treatment of osteoporosis: efficacy of combination of hormone replacement therapy with other antiresorptive agents," *J. Clin. Densitom.* 2000 Summer; 3(2):187–201.

Wysowski, D. K., G. W. Comstock, K. J. Helsing, H. L. Lasu, "Sex hormone levels in serum in relation to the development of breast cancer." *Am. J. Epidemiol.* 1987; 125:791–799.

Zeleniuch-Jacquotte, A., P. F. Bruning, J. M. G. Bonfrer, et al. "Relation of serum levels of testosterone and dehydroepiandrosterone sulfate to risk of breast cancer in postmenopausal women." *Am. J. Epidemiol.* 1997; 145:1030–1038.

Zuger, Abigail. "Challenge of Patch Drugs: Getting Under the Skin," *The New York Times* (August 17, 1999).

Zumoff, B., R. S. Rosenfeld, G. W. Strain, J. Levin, D. K. Fukushima, "Sex differences in the twenty-four-hour mean plasma concentrations of dehydroepiandrosterone (DHA) and dehydroepiandrosterone sulfate (DHAS) and the DHA:DHAS ratio in normal adults." *J. Clin. Endocrinol. Metab.* 1980; 51:330–333.

Zumoff, B., G. Strain, L. Miller, W. Rosner, "Twenty-four-hour mean plasma testosterone concentration declines with age in normal premenopausal women." *J. Clin. Endocrinol. Metab.* 1995; 80:1429–1430.